Basic Microcurrent Therapy Acupoint & Body Work Manual

Fourth Edition

Carolyn Wing Greenlee
with Dennis L. Greenlee, D.C., L.Ac.
& Thomas W. Wing, D.C., N.D., L.Ac.

Earthen
Vessel
Productions

Basic Microcurrent Therapy
Acupoint and Body Work Manual
©1995 Carolyn Wing Greenlee

Forth Edition
Feburary, 2018

ISBN: 978-1-887400-54-1

For professional guidance only
Notice: experimental use only

Our thanks to Dr. Ralph Alan Dale for his advice and editorial assistance

Cover: Daniel Worley and Stephanie Carol Del Bosco
Illustrations : Carolyn Wing Greenlee and Stephanie Carol Del Bosco
Layout: Carolyn Wing Greenlee and Daniel Worley

Published and distributed in the USA by
Earthen Vessel Productions, Inc.
Kelseyville, CA, USA
www.earthen.com

Dedication

To Daddy who pioneered it
To Dennis who ran with it
To the health professionals
      who have been catalyzed by my father's work,
      and the patients who enjoy the benefits of it all,

But especially to Jesus,
      Who designs every body
            and lovingly bestows life on each one

PREFACE

Our original manual was written in the late 1970s for those who attended our seminars on electro-acupoint therapy. My husband Dennis and I were teaching on the new art of non-needle acupoint therapy based on the discoveries of my father, Dr. Thomas W. Wing. Our book was specifically designed to help health professionals get the most out of Dr. Wing's Accu-O-Matic. We had no idea at that time that Dr. Wing's invention would start a revolution which would eventually become M.E.N.S. microcurrent.

Now, twenty years later, our desire is still that health professionals be able to use microcurrent confidently. This book is an overview, to give you the basics, the principles, and an idea of what microcurrent instruments can do.*

We hope you enjoy your adventure.

Carolyn Wing Greenlee

*Since there are now many instruments with different features and capabilities, not all of the information in this book may apply to your instrument.

Contents

Contraindications:

- Pregnant woman: Do not stimulate the Forbidden Points (LI4, SP6, ST36) or treat over the uterus.
- Heart problems: Do not treat over a pace maker or cross interferential over the heart.
- Do not treat over the area of metal implants. Exception: amalgams in teeth.
- Do not treat at the site of neuralgic pain, migraine headache, tic douloureux because it will irritate it.
- Do not treat over cancer.
- No specific contraindications for children.

Check your instrument instruction manual for other contraindications.

INSTRUMENTATION

Since there are now so many kinds of instruments of various vintages, the following is intended to be used as a guide. The controls described are applicable primarily to M.E.N.S.® microcurrent stimulators and search instruments, and similar clones and copies. Other instruments should be used with caution if they have higher voltages, currents and wave forms that could be hazardous. Health professionals should heed the precautions indicated by their instrument manufacturers.

CONTROLS

1. SEARCH/TREAT
    Not all microcurrent instruments have Search capabilities. Those that do will have a probe handle through which electrical conductance can be measured (see #10). Some instruments have a switch which changes the function of the main probe from Search to Treat. Other units are always on Search—treatment begins when the button on the handle is depressed. Search voltages are usually set by the manufacturer and cannot be changed. Check to see that the search current and voltage are such that the acupoint will not be altered on repeated or prolonged readings.

2. METER
    The meter indicates electrical resistance when the instrument is on SEARCH. The reading rises as resistance decreases. It lets you know contact is being made, and provides a direct energy readout for meridian balancing. The meter is coupled with sound; the pitch rises in proportion with increased conductance. Decreased resistance means increased conductance.

    The meters on Dr. Wing's original instruments were designed for Zero center for normal acupoints. His newer instruments have Zero to 100% meter scales that serve the dual purposes of search and conductance measurements for treatment current. Normal is 50% conductance.

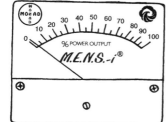

PERCENTAGE OF CONDUCTANCE																			
20	30	33	35	37	40	43	45	48	50	52	55	58	60	65	70	75	80	90	100

3. FREQUENCY - HERTZ (Hz)
Selects the speed of the wave cycle. Two full waves per second = 2 Hz (see "Hertz" p. 7). On instruments with two channels, you may have two frequency controls.

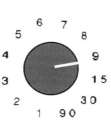

4. TREAT POLARITY SWITCH
"T" on the instrument stands for "Tsunami" in the bi-phasic mode. It is useful for the majority of functions. The "-" and "+" are mono-polar Tsunami waves, but are polarized for specific functions (see "Polarity" p. 8). On instruments with two channels, you may have two polarity controls.

5. WAVE SLOPE
Regulates the speed in which the wave ramps from 0–100%. Number 1, or Gentle, is the least disturbing and can be considered a "yin" approach, whereas #10, or Sharp, would be a "yang" approach. On instruments with two channels, you may have two wave slope controls.

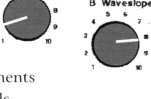

6. TIMER (seconds, minutes)
Regulates the length of the treatment cycle. For general body "Q" probe work, we treat for 5–10 seconds because the Tsunami Wave completes its bi-phasic cycles in multiples of 5 seconds.

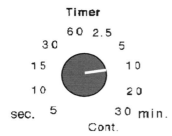

7. CURRENT LIMIT (μA=microamps)
Regulates the amount of power coming through the probe or pad. In Wing's instruments, current is selectable from 10 μA to 600 μA. On instruments with two channels, you may have two current limit controls.

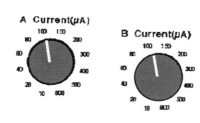

8. VOLTAGE OUTPUT
The higher the voltage, the deeper the penetration. For general work, use Medium setting. Don't use high voltage on acute conditions. Maximum 60 volts D.C. Pulsed 50% DUTY cycle (although voltages as low as 10 volts or even less will work, better longer lasting results are achieved with 60-volt instruments).

2

9. AUDIBLE SEARCH THRESHOLD

Threshold

Determines sound cutoff level. When it is turned completely to the left, sound will be on continually. Any time the search prob contacts the skin, the instrument will make more noise. The more to the right the knob is turned, the higher the signal has to be before the instrument will make noise.

10. AUDIBLE THRESHOLD INDICATOR LIGHT

When lit, it indicates that the sound is off. When the sound comes on, the light goes off. When the instrument is in operation, if the AUDIBLE SEARCH THRESHOLD is turned all the way to the right, the light will be on to let you know that the instrument is still on.

Example of use of Audible Threshold: If you wish to do Nogier's work and want to be notified of only those points whose readings, for example, exceed 50, you would do the following:

A. Turn the instrument to Search Mode.
B. Apply search probe to a point with sufficient pressure so that the meter reads as 50 (or whatever your chosen reading may be). Hold the steady reading, then
C. Turn the AUDIBLE SEARCH THRESHOLD knob clockwise until the sound barely goes off. The lighted LED indicates the sound is off.
D. Then turn the knob back slightly until the light and sound just come on again. The sound will correspond to the disappearance of the THRESHOLD light.
F. Now the meter needle will move as usual, but no sound will occur until the needle reaches and exceeds the Threshold setting. The light will also go off at this time.

Volume

11. VOLUME

Controls audible sound. Adjust to suit. Use Threshold control to mute the sound on standby if desired.

12. LED TREAT CURRENT INDICATOR LIGHT

Shows which polarity the treatment cycle is on. When the knob is on "T," the instrument is set to bi-phasic and there will be an alternation of high and low pitch and the lights will indicate + and - alternately. When the knob is on +, there will be a higher tone and only the + light will glow. When it is on -, there will be a tone lower in pitch from the +, and only the - light will glow. Brightness also indicates relative current flow. High current will show brighter.

13. LOW BATTERY INDICATION

Lo Batt

When lit, indicates need for replacement soon. Batteries should be removed to avoid damage from leakage. When replacing batteries, do not just replace a few. All the batteries should be replaced.

PROBES AND ELECTRODES

1. INDIFFERENT ELECTRODE

Serves as return and completes the circuit. Thus it must make contact with the patient's skin somewhere. It makes possible searching, treating, and evaluation. Two indifferent electrodes can be used together for increasing the energy of the patient, as well as for deep muscle work. Also called "hand-held electrode," "rod electrode," "roller," or "hand mass."

2. INDIFFERENT ELECTRODE HOLDER

Stainless steel hand mass fits into the holder. The holder also receives other probe tips such as the "Q", the auricular tips.

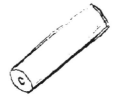

3. TREATMENT PROBE HANDLE

Receives probe tip. On instruments which measure electrical conductance, this is the receptor of the information. When the button is pressed, treatment begins.

4. PROBE TIPS

A large variety is available for different protocols. The "Q" holder invented by Wing is the most popular for general work. Metals such as stainless steel and brass are most common.

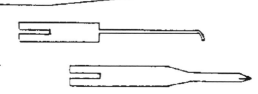

Wing's instruments now use threaded electrode tips which cannot be used with the older split-shank electrode holders, however the split-shank electrodes can be used with the threaded electrode holders.

Interferntial probes carry two frequencies and require special connectors.

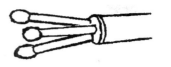 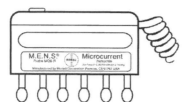

5. PADS
    Usually employed for longer durations and unattended protocols. The reusable ones are more economical, but must be sanitized between patients. Pads can be attached with adhesive gel or straps.

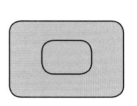 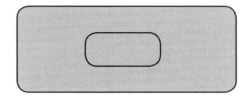

6. INDIFFERENT ELECTRODE WIRE
    The innerconnecting wire is used to connect the treatment probe and indifferent probe together.

7. CHANNELS
    A channel has two outputs, a negative and a positive. The output of instruments with one channel can be modified by Current, Frequency, Polarity, and Waveslope controls. All of the procedures in this manual except microcurrent interferential can be performed by a one-channel instrument. For microcurrent interferential, you need an instrument with two channels. A one-channel instrument with auxiliary outputs should not be confused with a two-channel instrument. Auxiliary outputs are not independent of the Main channel's control settings.

    Two-channel instruments have two sets of Main Treat Outputs: Channels A & B. There are independent Current, Frequency, Polarity and Waveslope controls for each channel with only the Volume and Timer controls being shared by both channels. Some older instruments have one universal Polarity and Waveslope control shared by both channels. Having a two-channel instrument gives you the capability of treating with microcurrent interferential as you can select a different frequency for each independent channel (see "Microcurrent Interferential" p. 23).

CURRENT, FREQUENCY (Hertz), WAVE FORM, POLARITY, AND WAVE SLOPE

CURRENT

A Microamps (μA), is one millionth of an amp, as opposed to a milliamp, which is one thousandth of an amp. Such a minute amount of current! Can it do any good? Here are a few thoughts: Robert Becker, M.D., reported that microcurrent was very close to being the same type of current as what flows through our bodies. Neil Spielholtz said, "My gut feeling is that the higher you go, the less beneficial the effect...I wouldn't be surprised to find that milliamps actually turn out to be counterproductive." The Arndt-Schutlz Law of the late 1800s stated: "Weak stimuli increase physiologic activity and very strong stimuli inhibit or abolish activity." Robert Picker, M.D., wrote, "Microamp stimulation has also been called 'biostimulation' or 'bioelectric therapy' because of its ability to stimulate cellular physiology and growth."

The body's response to the stimulation is determined by the strength of the stimulation, the method of stimulation, the time it's applied, the body's sensitivity to the stimulation and its ability to respond to it. When the stimulation is sufficient and reaches a specific level, the body will react to it. A very weak stimulation administered over a long period of time will eventually even create sedation.

Current settings determine the amount of electrical stimulation which is applied during the treatment cycle. Microamps in a range of from 20 to 100 μA is considered Slight. A range of 500 to 600 μA is considered Strong and might give the patient a little discomfort or a stinging sensation. In some acupuncture procedures, this is considered desirable, but most patients would prefer their treatments to be subsensory.

Additional research:

Cheng *et al* 1982 applied 500 μA to in vitro tissue and measured increases in the following: ATP production, 500%, protein synthesis, 70%, and cell transport, 40%.

Bourguigonon 1987, '88, '89 used similar research as Cheng *et al* for human tissue and reported enhanced tissue repair, protein, and DNA synthesis, improved insulin binding and increased intracellular calcium uptake.

Stanish 1988 applied μA current to surgically repaired Achilles tendon ruptures in athletes and found this group to heal 30% faster than the control group.

FREQUENCY (Hertz)

If this is one second, ——————— this is one Hertz. ∞ This is two Hertz. ∿∿ Hertz, also called "frequency," is the number of cycles per second. The fewer the cycles, the more stimulating the treatment. The more frequent the cycles per second, the more sedating. There are a number of different opinions on which frequencies are most effective, so you'll just have to see what works best for each situation. Don't be afraid to experiment.

Most researchers agree that the frequencies used in pain control are generally from 10 to 80 Hz and 300 Hz. These frequencies tend to bring about the best enkephalin response. Remember that the enkephalin response creates the most effective analgesia only while the current is turned on. Dr. Dennis Greenlee reports that, in pain control, the endorphin response is the most effective. It is accomplished in the frequency range of 1 to 10 Hz, with most authorities narrowing it to 4 to 7.

For auricular work, Dr. Nogier's system determines Hz according to the complexity of the tissue, whereas Dr. Robert Peshek, an holistic dentist, believes that 20 Hz provides the most long-lasting treatment. Dr. Wing, wanting to avoid having to change frequencies as per Nogier's work, chose 2.5 Hz as the universal frequency. He believes that 2.5 Hz will suffice in most cases if the correct points are chosen for treatment.

We have found that, since there are individual differences between patients and conditions, many times it is necessary to experiment with frequency changes when we do not achieve the expected or desired response. The following is a collection of frequencies which Dr. Greenlee has collected from colleagues, instructors, and researchers.

SUGGESTED FREQUENCIES

Balancing meridians, extremity points:	10 Hz
Body points and acupoints on body:	20 Hz
Muscle spasms and motor points:	1.2–2.5 Hz
Mucous membranes (hemorrhoids, inside nose, etc.):	.9–2.5 Hz
Skin, mechano nerve receptors, lymphatic tissue	300 Hz
Golgi tendon/spindle cell:	.1 Hz x length of muscle
Pain control:	Enkephalin response: 60–80 Hz and 300 Hz
	Endorphin response: 4–7 Hz
Auricular points:	20 Hz according to Peshek
	variable Hz according to Nogier
	2.5 Hz according to Wing

POLARITY (Directional Current)

Current can be set to negative, positive, or bi-phasic. Normally, bi-phasic (alternating DC pulsed current) will give a satisfactory response. It allows the body to make the choice of which polarity it wants. However, there are provocative experiments going on with mono polarity which may suggest innovative approaches to clinical problems.

In the 1980s, Robert Becker, M.D., experimented with regeneration of salamander limbs. He discovered that negative current applied to the blastema speeded up limb regrowth. He also discovered that humans are negatively charged in the extremities and positively charged along the central nervous systems, though the motor and sensory nerves are more negatively charged distally. In 1984, Becker and Selden reported the complete regeneration of the amputated fingertip of a child.

Negative current is antibacterial. Clinicians recommend using it around infected wounds, switching to positive and/or bi-phasic after the wound cultures clear. They report that negative current produces a stronger scar with elastin fibers that are oriented parallel to the skin surface as opposed to the fibers of an untreated scar, which are perpendicular.

In his article "Current Trends: Low-volt Pulsed Microamp Stimulation, Part II," Robert Picker, M.D. reports, "...many users believe that the positive pole has a more anti-inflammatory physiological effect, while the negative pole has a vasodialative effect, which can be helpful with muscle spasm and contracted scar tissue. The positive pole is used more often with acute injuries and the negative pole with chronic neuromuscular symptoms."

Positive current has a constrictive effect, decreases inflammation and sedates nerve irritation. It produces an acidic pH and augments the early closure of a wound. Dr. Greenlee says he remembers the uses of polarity by thinking of positive as ice which causes constriction and negative as heat which causes dispersal.

WAVE FORM

The usual form of a wave is curved like this: It is called a sine wave. Sine waves are like the waves of the ocean. They go back and forth, back and forth, ebb and flow. Negative, positive, negative, positive. Basically, they cancel each other out. If you took an impact wrench and tapped it once one direction and then tapped it once the other, you wouldn't get anything done.

Square waves are shaped like this: Notice that the waves oscillate negative and positive and counteract each other. A 4 Hz square wave looks like this: There are four oscillations in the space of one second.

The square wave fills the corners so it packs more energy than a sine wave. That is why Dr. Wing developed the Tsunami (pronounced "Sue-NAM-ee"), a synthetic square wave. It pulses steadily and continuously the same direction for two and a half seconds, like an impact wrench which taps the same direction--small taps adding up to a big force.

Biphasic Tsunami Waves begin in negative polarity and switch to positive.

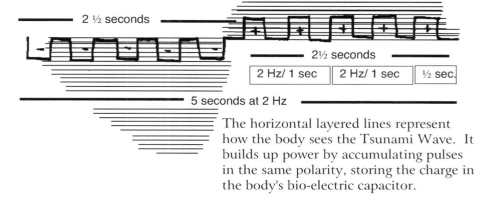

The square lines show what a complete bi-phasic 2 Hz Tsunami Wave looks like on an oscilloscope. Each Tsunami Wave cycle is 2½ seconds seconds regardless of frequency. A complete bi-phasic cycle takes 5 seconds. That is why Dr. Wing recommends treatments times of 5–10 seconds each.

The horizontal layered lines represent how the body sees the Tsunami Wave. It builds up power by accumulating pulses in the same polarity, storing the charge in the body's bio-electric capacitor.

WAVE SLOPE

Wave slope is designated in a range from Gentle to Sharp depending on how quickly the wave reaches its peak current. The diagram to the right shows a Tsunami Wave with a sharp wave slope. Under it is a Tsunami Wave with a gentle wave slope.

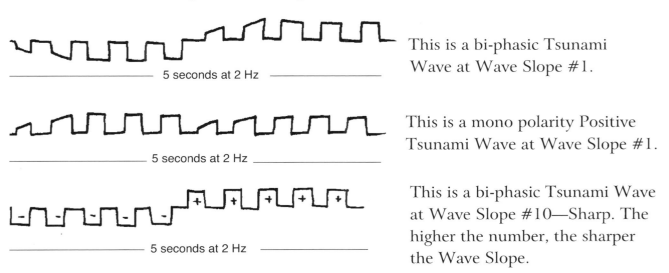

This is a bi-phasic Tsunami Wave at Wave Slope #1.

This is a mono polarity Positive Tsunami Wave at Wave Slope #1.

This is a bi-phasic Tsunami Wave at Wave Slope #10—Sharp. The higher the number, the sharper the Wave Slope.

Wave slope selection is important for successful tonification or sedation. For tonification, the wave slope should be soft and comfortable. In sedation, it should be stronger and slightly uncomfortable. Use Gentle for acute conditions and Sharp for pain control. Use Moderate for chronic complaints, functions, and all standard conditions.

9

PREPARING THE "Q" PROBE

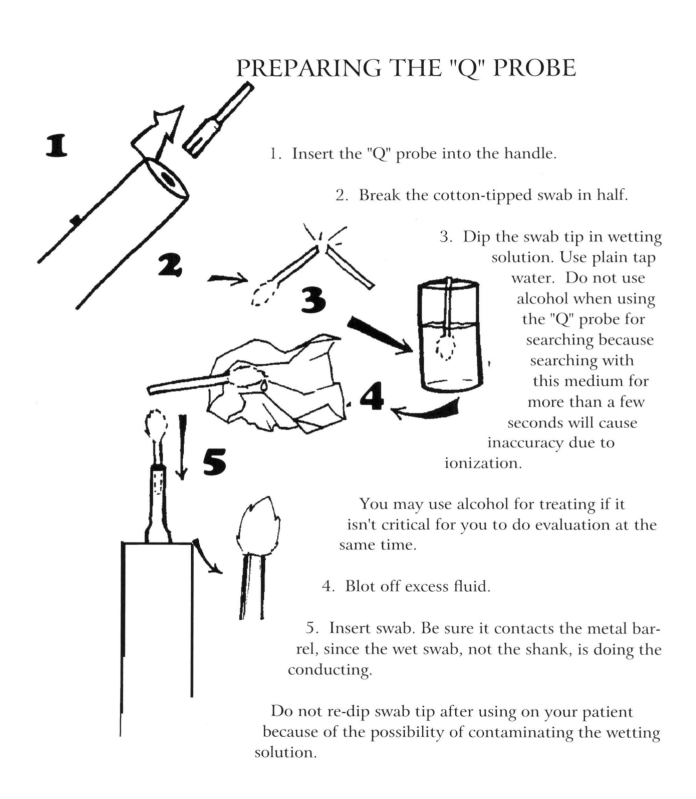

1. Insert the "Q" probe into the handle.

2. Break the cotton-tipped swab in half.

3. Dip the swab tip in wetting solution. Use plain tap water. Do not use alcohol when using the "Q" probe for searching because searching with this medium for more than a few seconds will cause inaccuracy due to ionization.

You may use alcohol for treating if it isn't critical for you to do evaluation at the same time.

4. Blot off excess fluid.

5. Insert swab. Be sure it contacts the metal barrel, since the wet swab, not the shank, is doing the conducting.

Do not re-dip swab tip after using on your patient because of the possibility of contaminating the wetting solution.

BODY WORK

BODY WORK

DIFFERENCES OF OPINION

If there's one thing practitioners know, it's that patients are unique individuals and their problems rarely fit the exact descriptions in the books. Practitioners are individuals as well. Four master acupuncturists evaluating the same patient might come up with four entirely different approaches to the problem. That is why healing is an art.

In this chapter, Dr. Wing's approach to body pattern treatment is presented, followed by a chapter by Dr. Dennis Greenlee, another doctor of chiropractic and acupuncture. Their approaches and procedures differ, though both have had good success with their patients. We offer them here together that you may benefit from the knowledge and experience of both.

ELECTRICAL CURRENT, SKIN RESISTANCE, AND NON-NEEDLE ACUPUNCTURE

Q: In electro acupoint therapy, do I have to be exactly on the acupoint to be effective?

A: No. In acupuncture, the placement of needles is crucial. Wing compares acupuncture to golf. In needle acupuncture, every stroke must be a Hole in One. A near-miss doesn't count. In contrast, electrical stimulation is like hitting the golf ball on a funnel-like slope with the hole at the lowest point so every shot is a Hole in One. As long as the ball is anywhere near the target, it will drop into the hole.

Skin has a specific resistance to electrical current, but, at the site of each acupoint, the resistance is lower. This is how electrical current, flowing like water down the path of least resistance, finds the acupoint. With your instrument on Search, you can draw the "Q" probe along the skin near the location of the acupoint. When the pitch and meter reading rises, you've found an active point.

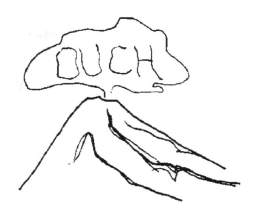

When an area of the body has been traumatized, myriads of acupoints pop up in the area to let off some of the stress—much as volcanoes permit Earth to let off steam. This is one reason that, in body point pattern work, most likely there will be a reactive point wherever you place your probe. Dr. Yoshio Nakatani, one of the first pioneers of electro therapy, called them "Reactive Permiable Points" (RPP). They are not true acupoints. These extra points tend to disappear as the area returns to normal.

PATTERNS

These are basic patterns with many applications. They can be used in wound healing, pain control, for relaxation, or to promote healing.

SHOTGUN

As the name implies, make contacts all through the area of complaint. Keep the probe on each spot until after its treatment cycle has ended. For pain control, use settings of 7–10 Hz. To move fluid or bring energy to the area, use .6–10 Hz for 5–10 seconds.

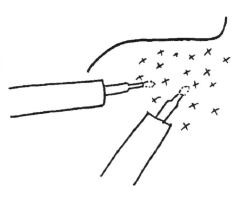

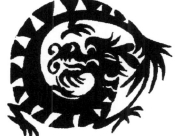

CIRCLE THE DRAGON

1. Treat clockwise starting at 12 o'clock, making contact at intervals corresponding to the face of the clock every 3 hours.

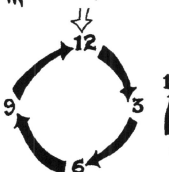 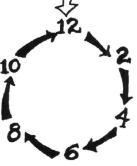 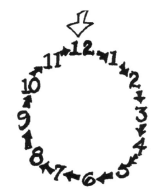

2. If the condition is more severe, treat points at intervals corresponding to the two-hour positions or at hourly positions or circle the perimeter of the area of dysfunction.

To speed up the treatment, use 2 "Qs " starting with one at 12 o'clock and the other at 6 o'clock.

To *really* speed things up, use the MQ-2 probe which has 2 "Qs" per probe.

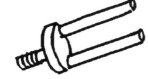

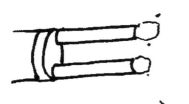

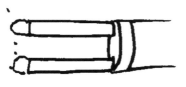

Hold probes perpendicular to surface

Circle a bruised area, or a swollen one.

Do not treat directly on an ulcer. Treat around the area using 5–20 Hz. Stimulations may be spaced fairly closely.

For hemorrhoids, use four points around GV 20 (top of the head) ending with GV 20. Use 20 Hz, 100 μA, 5–10 seconds. For really bad hemorrhoids, circle the hemorrhoid itself, touching the line of demarcation at intervals of one-eighth of an inch. Use .9 Hz for 5–10 seconds per stimulation. Finish with GV 20 at 20 Hz for 1 minute.

For Plantars Warts, circle around the edge at 10 Hz, using 100 μA for 5–10 seconds.

For noses and ear canals, press the Q-tip firmly against the surface being treated. Overlap stimulations slightly. Use lowest microamps. Treat nose at 20 Hz or 80 Hz. Treat ears at 20 Hz or 2 ½ Hz.

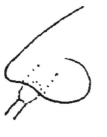

Eyes and sinus—or dispersal, treat in a small pattern, then a larger one. To increase energy, do the larger circle first, then the smaller. Use 10 Hz for 10 sec. with μA less than 100. Patients usually experience a light show—flashing spots of bright light.

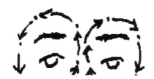

We've never found it to be detrimental to the patient. If the patient feels sting-ing at the points of contact, reduce the level of current. Do not treat *through* the eyes.

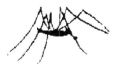

For insect bites, use two "Q"s. Make contact directly on the bite. Make sure the cotton swab is quite wet. Circle the Dragon using at least four points about a quarter inch from center. For group bites, place the indifferent "Q" electrode (the one that does not search) at center of group and circle using at least six points about a quarter inch outside the group. If there is no relief in ten minutes, repeat using more points.

Dr. Greenlee uses Circle the Dragon with ulcers and other open wounds. Some-times he uses the clock pattern around the area; sometimes he uses the indifferent "Q" electrode in the center and circles around it. Note: When dealing with an open lesion, sterilize the probes before and after treatment.

We usually keep our instrument Current setting in a medium range. On sensitive ar-eas or places of great dysfunction, use the lowest setting possible. When using a metallic contact such as the indifferent hand mass or the ball-tip probe for therapy, use the low-est setting to avoid stinging. You can also keep the metal electrodes wet with ultrasound gels. With a moist contact, stinging is minimized. For the indifferent hand mass, a wet paper towel over the treating surfaces helps (unless you're using it in ways which make wet paper towels impractical).

The Tsunami Wave supercharges the point so, at higher current levels, even with the "Q" probe, the patient may feel an extra sensation (like a little bite) at the end of the treatment cycle. This is not terribly painful, but you might alert your patient to the pos-sibility. The more dysfunctional a point is, the more likely it is to be sore to the touch, and the more sensation the patient will feel. Try reducing the current, especially when treating with all-metal electrodes such as the auricular probes.

FLOW OF ENERGY

Energy is always in motion. It is known by its effects. A breeze that stops is no longer a breeze. So it is with energy. In the body, energy flows through twelve major channels, which are called meridians. As long as this energy is unobstructed and balanced, health remains.

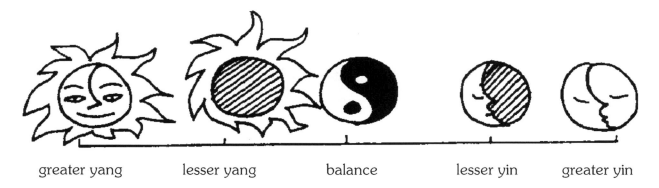

greater yang   lesser yang   balance   lesser yin   greater yin

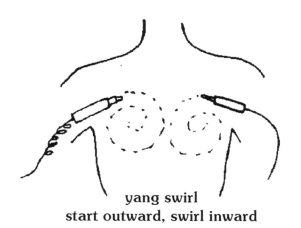

yang swirl
start outward, swirl inward

The Chinese see the principles of yin and yang in relationship to one another operating throughout all of life, and particularly in terms of the functions of the body. The words Yin and Yang may be confusing and intimidating to Western minds, but they may be very helpful in providing another approach in dealing with health problems. These brief descriptions may make these terms more accessible.

Some yang: warm, dry, yellow, pain, excessive, vertical, external, aggressive, superficial, positive, male, narrow, straight, acute, active

Some yin: cool, wet, blue, numbness, deficient, horizontal, internal, passive, deep, negative, female, wide, curved, chronic, static

Though all female is yin, not all yin is female. Not all yang is male. And not all yin is bad. With our Western yang minds, we tend to think that negative means undesirable, that inactivity is a waste of time, and that passivity is the way to lose. But negative ions actually feel good, rest is restorative, and often you gain more life by giving it away. Also, as we Californians know, all sunny days makes for a water shortage. Yin and yang are descriptions, not value judgments.

Energy is always in flux. We inhale (yin), exhale (yang), eat (yin), excrete (yang), wake (yang), sleep (yin). Energy ebbs (yin) and flows (yang): we take it in (yin), we give it out (yang). The dynamic must remain—an even exchange—otherwise we get overheated (yang) or drained (yin), congested (yang) or dissipated (yin). Blockages create energy jams. Chi (life force) backs up behind the dam and becomes pain. Lack of Chi becomes numbness, coldness. Absolute Yin is death.

SWIRLING THE DRAGON

Swirling the Dragon is a spiral form of Circling the Dragon made possible by Wing's adaptation of microcurrent to the Chinese pattern.

1. Concentrate energy in an area by swirling towards it. This also improves circulation. It is a yang procedure.

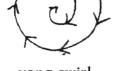

yang swirl   **yin swirl**

2. Disperse energy by swirling away from the area of complaint. This is also useful to break up congestion and relieve pain. It is a yin procedure.

3. For pumping action, swirl inward, then outward. If you want to increase energy, swirl inward again. To decrease, end with a swirl outward.

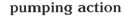

pumping action

4. To increase the energy in an area, treat towards the midline of the body. To decrease energy, treat away from the midline.

5. Try sequential stimulation for dispersal. Follow the meridians, if you know them, for added effectiveness. Meridians flow from the lowest number to the highest (see bottom of p. 59). Move with the energy flow to tonify, against to sedate.

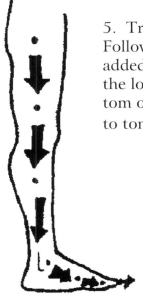

yin effect

For swirling procedures, treat with one "Q" probe while your patient holds the indifferent electrode in one hand, or use two "Q" probes, one behind the other in a yin or yang direction. Because the current flows between the probes, having the points of contact near each other helps direct the chi in the direction you choose.

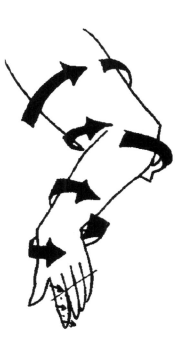

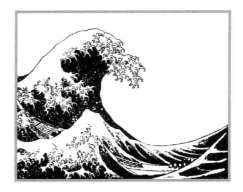

T.E.S.T.
Transcutaneous Electro-Stimulation Tsunami

We feel that T.E.S.T. goes beyond mere pain control. We believe that it actually triggers healing due to the nature of the Tsunami Wave with its directed polarity (see Wave Form p. 8). Any of the proceeding body patterns can be adapted to T.E.S.T. by fitting the indifferent electrode holder with a "Q" probe and moving it to a position which causes the electrical current to pass through to the area being treated.

cross section

T.E.S.T. PATTERNS

T.E.S.T. THROUGH
Place one "Q" electrode on the side opposite to the one being treated. Use the shotgun technic or Circle the Dragon.

T.E.S.T. AROUND
Use the swirling pattern with the "Q" probes on opposite sides. These procedures are used in pain control. Swirl the Dragon for greater effectiveness—outward for dispersal (yin), inward for strengthening (yang).

T.E.S.T. ASSOCIATE POINTS
With one "Q" probe on either side of the spine, treat the Associate Points (two parallel lines on both sides of the spine, following the Bladder meridian—see p. 98) in a downward direction. Use it for spinal injuries, post fractures, back sprain, and as a general tonic.

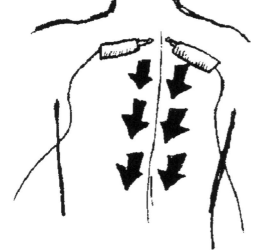

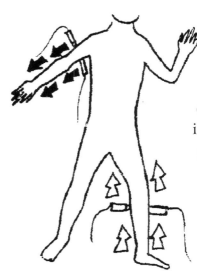

SEQUENTIAL T.E.S.T.

Using your knowledge and understanding of the direction of energy flow in the body, treat the body in either yin or yang directions for energy increase or pain control. For additional pain control, treat the Associate Points sequentially, moving the energy away from the area of injury and pain. Begin near the spine and treat in parallel lines in a downward direction: A, then B, then C.

ETR
(Enhancing Tissue Repair)

Cells die all the time, yet dysfunction in an area continues. New cells do not return to normal. Instead, they perpetuate the condition of dysfunction. The drawing to the left shows the basic biochemical feedback mechanism which illustrates the hypothesis that

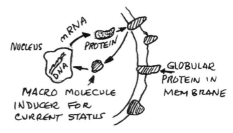

membrane structure is determined by the current genetic activity of a cell. Globular proteins (*e.g.*, enzymes) in the membrane maintain the current genetic activity. The drawing to the right represents Wing's belief that a new inducer may be liberated from another in-

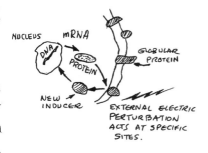

dependent membrane globular protein under the action of an external (electrical perturbation, which thus provides a new feedback loop. This may make possible changes in information transmitted to the nucleus, which could trigger repair activities.

ETR is Wing's procedure of using two "Q's" to accelerate tissue repair. The Tsunami Wave, with its cumulative power, is able to break down the ohmic barrier of normal skin, allowing the stimulating signal to pass through in sufficient quantity to trigger tissue repair with efficacy not previously obtained.

1. Align the injured tissue between the "Q" probes, positioning the probes along the area of injured tissue so that the current is directed through the tissue area needing repair.
2. Press the Treat button to start the treatment cycle.
3. Wait for each treatment cycle to finish before moving to the next location.

EMR
(Enhancing Muscle Repair)

The EMR theory is that the electrical reprogramming signal (described under ETR p. 19) must pass between the Z lines of the sarcomere. There seems to be a "venetian blind" effect. Unless the signal current is injected perpendicularly to the muscle fibers, it cannot pass through the opening in the Actin. Dr. Wing believes the proper triggering of the sarcomere will result in a normal resting contractile unit. This is why it's so important to follow the exact striations of the muscles.

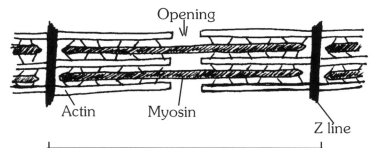

This drawing shows the contractile mechanism of normal skeletal muscles.

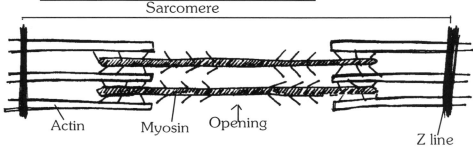

This drawing shows a stretched muscle. Notice that the gap in the Actin is much wider.

1. Starting at the origin of the muscle, contact the muscle fibers at a perpendicular angle, lifting the fibers between the "Q" probes.

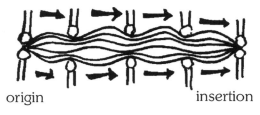

2. Follow the length of the muscle, spacing the stimulations about one half inch apart until they reach the insertion of the muscle. Space them closer if the condition is more severe.

If needed, consult a muscle chart for accuracy of direction.

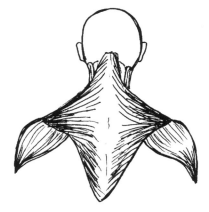

GOLGI TENDON & SPINDLE CELLS

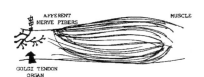

The Golgi tendon organ is the governing reflex found within the tendon at the attachments of the muscles. It prevents the muscle from being overstretched. Spindle cells are in the belly of the muscle. They monitor the strength of the muscle contraction. They also will relax or tonify the muscle.

GOODHEART/WING GOLGI TENDON TECHNIC

Goodheart theorizes that his technic refastens the anchor points of the muscle tendon. He believes that hard mechanical pressure helps reaffirm this connection just as pressing over the magnetic catch of a gapy refrigerator door reestablishes a magnetic bond. Wing substitutes M.E.N.S. microcurrent with mild mechanical pressure and applies Goodheart's procedure as described below.

1. Place selected muscle in a stretch to activate Golgi tendon organ. Using 8 to 10 ounces of pressure, press with probes directed at the origin and insertion of the muscle in a direction away from the belly of the muscle.

To use spindle cells to release, use muscle fibers in the belly. Press with probes directed towards each other. Use moistened cotton-tiped swabs (wooden or plastic-shanked swabs may be necessary). To strengthen the muscle with spindle cells, direct the probes in the belly of the muscle away from each other.

2. Treat at .6 Hz at 50–100 μA or to tolerance of patient for 10–15 seconds per stimulation.

3. Repeat this on each group of muscles. For the trapezius, for example, use three spots—one for the upper, one for the middle, and one for the lower Trap.

4. For a different approach, stroke the muscle using a longer treatment cycle time, or with the timer on Continuous.

NOTICE: Dr. Wing does not recommend this technic on inflammatory muscles since muscle spasms may result. He suggests EMR as the first therapy, attempting to normalize the muscle rather than merely refasten it.

NEW MULTIPLE PROBE
ELECTRODE ADAPTATIONS

Wing has developed the MQ-2 swab electrode holder which features two standard swabs spaced about half an inch apart. The MQ-2 allows the stimulating signal to cover a much larger area than with the single "Q". Use two MQ-2s when performing ETR and EMR technics or with Circling or Swirling the Dragon or T.E.S.T.. This probe is particularly effective on small surfaces such as fingers.

You may also use a combination of one MQ-2 on the treatment handle and an indifferent rod electrode on the opposition handle. While the patient holds the stainless steel hand mass, treat with the MQ-2 through the fingers wrapped around the hand mass.

GETTING INTERFERENTIAL
WHILE USING JUST ONE FREQUENCY

The dual "Q" electrode provides two pathways rather than a single one. The illustration on the left shows the path of current from one set of opposing probes. The one on the right shows the paths of two. When two apertures are used, the difference in the travel time of the current passing through the tissue will result in different phases. Where they meet, they interfere with each other, thus creating a slight interferential phase shift with one frequency.

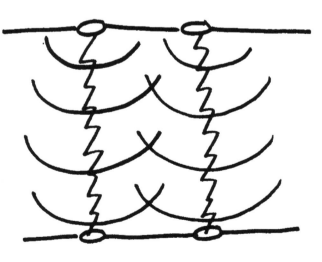

MICROCURRENT INTERFERENTIAL

Because interferential requires some planning and understanding, many practitioners have decided it's too much trouble. While it's true that the procedures are more demanding than the "point and shoot" type, the potentials for healing are well worth the effort. This section contains some pointers which may help clear things up for you.

Unless there are two different frequencies and the pads or probes which carry them are positioned so that those frequencies cross (creating interference) within the body, you don't have true interferential. But if you position them right, you have created four frequencies which the body can use--the two injected frequencies, and their sum and difference. This is, of course, assuming you're using microcurrent interferential, not high frequency milliampere interferential.

A Frequency

.3

B Frequency

.9

To perform interferntial, you need a two-channel instrument, each with one red port and one black port. Insert a red and a black lead into the A side. Then insert a red and a black into the B side.

Set the A side to one frequency (such as .3 or 3 Hz) and the B side to another (such as .9 or 9 Hz).

Then place the Red A pad on one side of the body (such as the front) and the Red B pad spaced away from the Red A pad. Place the Black A pad opposing the Red B pad (on the back of the body), and the Black B pad opposite the Red A pad. The current flows between the Red + and the Black - electrodes. Thus the currents will cross each other as shown in the diagram cross section. Pad times run usually a minimum of five minutes to as long as desired. Most use 15 to 30 minutes unattended. Current is usually about 100 to 300 μA.

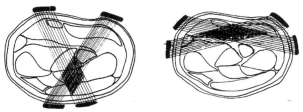

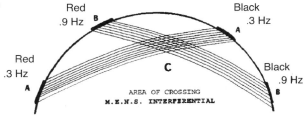

Red
.9 Hz B

Black
.3 Hz A

Red
.3 Hz
A

Black
.9 Hz
B

C

AREA OF CROSSING
M.E.N.S. INTERFERENTIAL

Current may be "steered" by pad placement. The cross-hatched area is the site of interferential activity.

Illustration above is from Dr. Wing's article "Interferential Therapy: How It Works and What's New," *Chiropractic Economics,* May/June, 1992. The ones on the left are from "The Power Is in Your Hands, Part II," *Chiropractic Economics,* March/April, 1988.

PROBE INTERFERENTIAL

Interested in the efficacy of interferential and wanting to adapt the principles to probe procedures, Wing developed the 3 D interferential probe. It has three sockets. A "Q" probe can be fitted into each one, making possible increased aperture injection of current. If two "Qs" are desired, the sockets are designed so the operator can chose wider or more narrow spacing of the probes.

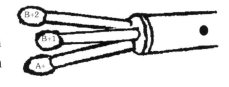

In this application, the probes deliver two currents instead of one. The opposition probe carries the two return electrodes. Each probe has its usual current, but the two frequencies are different. This produces the interferential or "beat" frequencies at the crossing of the two currents within the tissues.

The treatment probe handle has three openings, all of which carry the positive current. Channel A is left of the treatment button. The other two openings are B. The opposition probe carries the negative. You may use two "Qs" with variable spacing as shown below, or three, with the B channel split (the power at the injection is divided between the two Bs). Stimulation time is usually from 5 to 30 seconds per spot. Current is 40–100 μA. Make sure the currents cross as shown in the diagram above.

The illustrations below show the probable paths of the two separate currents as they cross within the body tissues with perpendicular placement of the electrodes. The three "Q" probes allow the operator the choice of variable spacing.

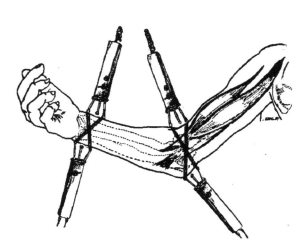

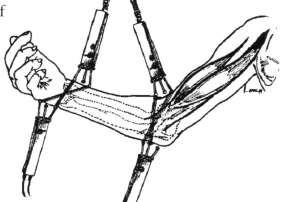

Illustrations from Dr. Wing's article "New Breakthrough in Multiple "Q" Electrodes" published in *Chiropractic Economics* March/April, 1989

PROBE INTERFERENTIAL MQ-6

Dennis L. Greenlee, D.C., L.Ac.

The MQ-6 probe is an advancement on the 3 D probes in that, instead of one cross-pattern interferential stimulation, there are three. These encompass a larger area of simultaneous stimulation. The frequencies used are the same as with all the other interferential procedures, but the effectiveness is greatly multiplied because of the electrical "chaos" which is developed within the area being treated.

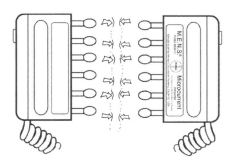

The MQ-6 has a variety of procedural advantages because of the number of probes being used on each stimulation. Because of the spring-retraction of each probe, the MQ-6 can be used over irregular surfaces. In treating with EMR, larger contact with each muscle is accomplished, reducing the number of contacts needed to cover an area. Treating with ETR, larger surfaces can be contacted with the advantage of interferential stimulation.

When interferential is not desired, probes can be positioned where they do not face each other so that there is no crossing of currents. Probe frequencies can be set individually; you can set them both to the same frequency. This also takes them out of interferential mode. You can stroke down the back, one MQ-6 on each side, or front and back simultaneously, or comb down an area with one probe following the other.

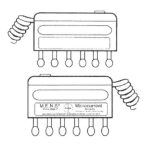

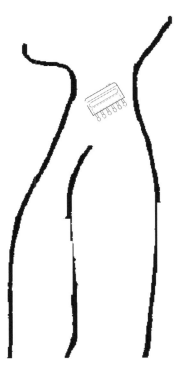

Since each probe contains both positive and negative current, you can use a single probe to stroke over large surface areas to help move lymphatic fluids.

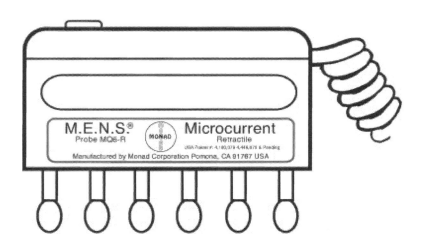

25

The MQ-6 and 3D Interferential Probes

When two different frequencies intersect or "interfere" with one another, the sum and difference of those frequencies will create two more frequencies. This is the principal of interferential. See example below:

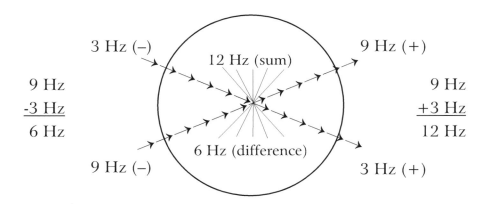

Traditional Interferential uses the principle of mixing a 4000 Hz and a 4001–5000 Hz frequency to generate the single desired frequency of 1–1000 Hz. These high frequencies are useless in therapy, but by mixing two frequencies, the minus frequency can be created in the desired range.

With microcurrent interferential, four frequencies can be available to the body: the two injected frequencies plus their sum and difference. This is because microcurrent is very similar to the body's own energy and thus the body does not resist the minute but effective stimulation.

Pad and Probe Interferential

Not only do the Monad two channel instruments offer you microcurrent interferential with pads, they also have the unique capabilities of interferential with probes. With the 3D or MQ-6 Interferential Probes, your treatments are not confined to one area for 15 minutes. You are able to move around the body treating more areas in less time. For example, you can use a creeping or combing technique to treat a whole extremity, flooding the area with four therapeutic frequencies in just over a minute.

The MQ-6 has unique retractable electrodes that conform to the contours of various body surfaces to insure even current flow, stable conductance and comfort. MQ-6s are effective when treating muscles, larger joints, the spine, knee, elbow, neck and shoulder. 3D probes are effective in the application to TMJs and small joints such as fingers and hands, wrists, ankles, feet, and toes.

3D Interferential Probe

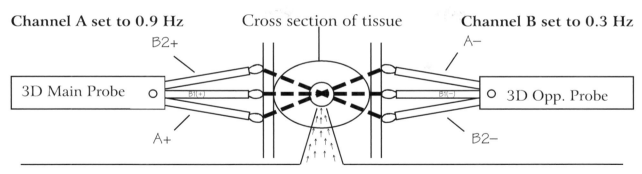

Channel A set to 0.9 Hz   Cross section of tissue   **Channel B set to 0.3 Hz**

B2+   A−

3D Main Probe   B1(+)   B1(−)   3D Opp. Probe

A+   B2−

Active Useful Frequencies: 0.9 Hz, 0.3 Hz, 1.2 Hz (the sum of A & B) & 0.6 Hz (the difference of A & B)
Note: Current flow will vary depending on underlying areas of tissue, muscle, bone and vessels.

MQ-6 Interferential Probe

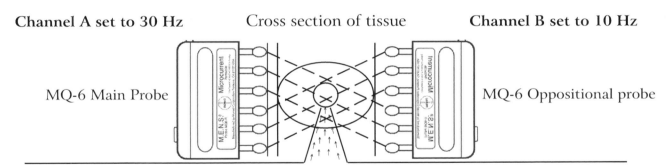

Channel A set to 30 Hz   Cross section of tissue   **Channel B set to 10 Hz**

MQ-6 Main Probe   MQ-6 Oppositional probe

Active Useful Frequencies: 30 Hz, 10 Hz, 40 Hz (the sum of A & B) & 20 Hz (the difference of A & B)
Note: Current flow will vary depending on underlying areas of tissue, muscle, bone and vessels.

MQ-6 Retractability

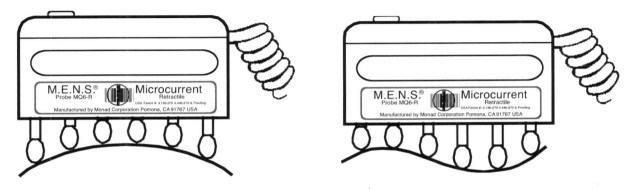

BODY WORK PROCEDURE

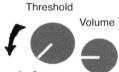

1.   Set up the instrument according to directions.

      A.   Audible Search Threshold turned completely to the left.

      B.   Set volume at a comfortable level.

      C.   Select frequency, treatment time, and current levels.

2.   Ask your patient to indicate and evaluate his pain, range of motion, etc..

3.   Select area to treat and decide on pattern to use (Circle, Swirl, T.E.S.T., ETR, Golgi, etc.).

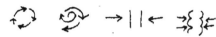

4.   Prepare Q-tip.

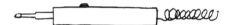

5.   Warn first-time patient about possible stinging. Should there be any unpleasant sensations, remove the probe right away and reduce the current. Keep under $100 \, \mu A$. Use lowest current that is still effective.

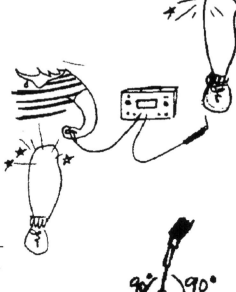

6.   Place the indifferent electrode in the hand of the patient corresponding to the side being treated.

7.   Make a firm contact with the "Q" probe approximately perpendicular to the point being treated.

8.   If your instrument has a search mode, you may search for hot points which will be indicated by a rise on the meter and in the pitch of the search tone. If your instrument does not have a search mode, or if you want to treat without looking for the most reactive points, simply make contact with the skin, press the treatment button on the probe handle, and hold steady until the treatment cycle has been completed.

9. When you have maximum response from the point, proceed to the next point to be treated (see E-PAT below).

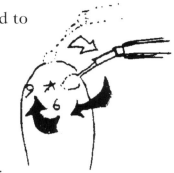

10. When you have completed your procedure, ask your patient to reevaluate.

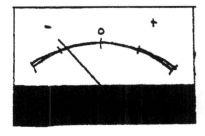

11. If there is insufficient relief, you may want to try Ear-Ricular points, a different body work approach, or meridian balancing.

E-PAT
(Evaluating Point After Treatment)

It is now possible, after five thousand years, to know whether you have "broken through" at the acupoint—whether it requires additional stimulation, or if the point is dysfunctional. (This is for instruments with Search capabilities only.)

1. When the treatment probe contacts the skin, the meter reading and the pitch of the search tone will rise. This represents the electrical resistance of the skin at this point.

2. On older instruments with needle-type meters, when you press the Treat button, the needle will drop into the range to the left of the initial reading and the instrument will make a sound which modulates (faster or slower according to the Frequency setting). On Monad M.E.N.S. instruments, the needle will drop and rise several times. The high readings indicate how much of the charge the body is accepting. If you have a Monad M.E.N.S. instrument with an LED meter, the lights will flash from the left to the right several times. The high readings indicate how much of the charge the body is accepting. DO NOT MOVE THE PROBE.

3. After the treatment cycle has been completed, the meter reading and pitch will rise. If the point has accepted the full charge, the reading will rise rapidly, then settle back slowly as the discharge from the acupoint dissipates. You can determine if the acupoint has accepted the full charge by noting whether the reading swings past the initial reading. The faster and higher it swings, the more energy has been accepted. (We taught our patients what the readings meant. They used to root for the meter.)

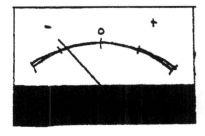 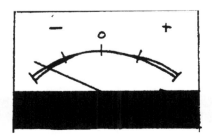 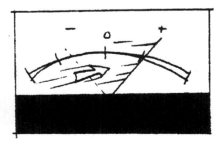

On instruments with a sensitivity switch:

~ If the original reading is in the excessive range, you won't be able to determine whether you broke through. Switch the sensitivity to a lower setting so the initial reading will appear on the meter in a more manageable range.

~ If the patient's energy is so low that you can hardly get a reading, switch the sensitivity to a higher setting so you can see a normal amount of conductance when the point is contacted.

4. If the first stimulation cycle does not create a breakthrough, repeat the treatment without moving the probe. If you try four or five times with little response, try another frequency (hands and feet like 10 Hz).* Or you may have reached an area of tremendous edema or energy blockage. The current may be too low or contact resistance too high preventing the current from flowing easily. Increase microamps or pressure (depending on what you're treating). You can also apply the principle of opposites and treat the same point on the opposite side. Then return to the original side and try it again.

~ Sometimes there is not enough conductance through the probe because the "Q" probe has dried out. Make sure it stays wet and that the moisture makes contact with the metal shaft of the probe.

~ Sometimes there is so much blockage that the point can't fire through. If it doesn't change after you've tried everything and hit it four or five times, it probably isn't going to. This is not uncommon when the areas of complaint are very old (such as arthritis). Check next time you treat. Microcurrent has a cumulative effect and the points should be easier to break through as balance is restored to the rest of the body.

---

* If the reading keeps getting lower, stop treating that point. You may be getting a sedation effect.

W.E.T.
Wing Electro Therapy
by Dennis L. Greenlee, D.C., L.Ac.

Microcurrent, like chiropractic or acupuncture, is not a panacea, but a useful modality when properly applied. These procedures may be used as a primary treatment modality, however I feel they are best utilized as adjunctive or as combined treatment with chiropractic, acupuncture, homeopathic, or naturopathic procedures. In my practice, I use all of the above.

To determine the approach to use with transcutaneous stimulation, it is necessary to determine the type of problem which the patient presents.

A. Is it an acute traumatic injury to a joint or to the muscles and soft tissue?
B. Is it an acute organic condition?
C. Is it a chronic structure or post traumatic condition?
D. Is it a combination of any of the above?

When the condition is acute with swelling, inflammation, pain, and immobility, the most effective initial treatment is transcutaneous stimulation—first treating the site of injury with T.E.S.T., ETR, or EMR stimulation. After treating the area of complaint, treat the dermatome innervation and trace the meridian and adjacent area or opposite dermatome or meridian area for trigger points.

I use T.E.S.T. immediately following any manipulative procedure in the area of the affected spine—treating each side of the spinous processes. Then I do ETR to the supportive and affected muscles of the area.

I have also found Wing's ETR effective in the treatment of sprains, strains, contusions, and bruises as well as for bites and burns. Consider the use of ETR whenever there is a need for serous fluid movement, and wherever you wish to increase circulation.

31

Golgi tendon and spindle cell treatment, discovered by Goodheart and electrified by Wing, is used in areas of decreased mobility where there are hypertonic or hypotonic muscles. However, when working in areas with swelling and acute pain, ETR should precede the treatment or the treatment should be delayed for several days. When Golgi tendon or spindle cell procedures are used too soon, you may aggravate the complaint.

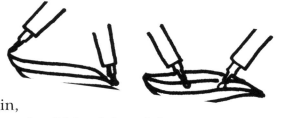

The treatment of acute organic disorders requires diligence in locating the organ or organs of involvement. You need to consider the patient's symptoms, the degree of involvement, and the energetic relationship of the organs to the body. It is necessary to use a traditional diagnostic approach to determine and locate the problems associated with the symptoms. To help locate the problems, examine the Associate and Alarm Points, since most organs refer pain and tenderness to those areas.

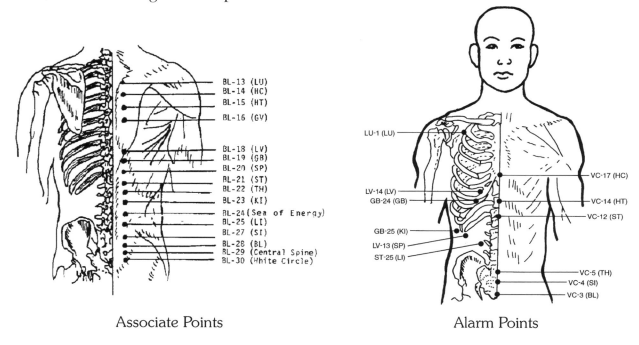

Associate Points   Alarm Points

For doctors with instruments capable of doing meridian balance, it is useful to take meridian readings to note the energetic relationships in the condition.

Some doctors have instruments which are capable of measuring specific organ points. This should be done whenever possible.

TRANSCUTANEOUS ELECTRO-STIMULATION PROCEDURES

After analysis and diagnosis of the patient's condition, it is necessary to determine the type of treatment procedure and the possible combinations of electrodes to be used. Possible combinations are as follows:

1. Two metal hand-held electrodes
2. One metal hand-held indifferent electrode and one treatment probe
3. One rubber pad and one treatment "Q" probe
4. Two treatment probes
5. Double pads

TREATMENT APPLICATIONS

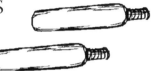

1. Two hand-held electrodes

A. For patients who demonstrate general low energy within the body, in the upper or lower portions of the body, or have generalized lower energy between left and right sides, this treatment can be used to flood the body with energy. The patient holds one electrode in each hand, or make contact with one foot and one hand, or with both feet.

Hz:	10–20 Hz
Microamps:	600 μA or to patient's tolerance
Wave Slope:	Gentle, slow rise
Time:	10 minutes

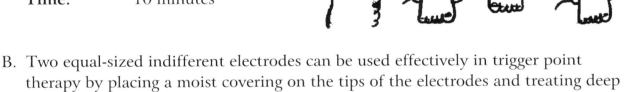

B. Two equal-sized indifferent electrodes can be used effectively in trigger point therapy by placing a moist covering on the tips of the electrodes and treating deep muscle trigger points, and/or large muscle trigger points.

Hz:	4–7 Hz
Microamps:	100 μA
Wave Slope:	Sharp, quick rise to peak current
Time:	Until maximum response

2. One hand-held (indifferent) electrode and one treatment "Q" probe
   Patient holding the hand-held electrode and operator using the probe

   A. Pattern #1: Treatment of acupuncture points

   Use when utilizing formula treatments with specific acupuncture points, trigger points, and electro-reactive points, and with specific auricular points.

Hz:	10 Hz for extremities
	20 Hz for body
Microamps:	20 μA to patient's tolerance
Wave Slope:	Moderate to Sharp
Time:	15–20 seconds

   B. Pattern #2: Shotgun

   When treating a small affected area, treat at random with the treatment probe.

Hz:	20 Hz
Microamps:	100 μA
Wave Slope:	Moderate to Sharp
Time:	5–15 seconds

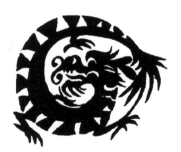

   C. Pattern #2: Surrounding the Dragon

   Choose the area of complaint (such as an eye, sinus, a bite, or contusion) and treat around the edge of complaint.

Hz:	20 Hz
Microamps:	100 μA
Wave Slope:	Moderate to Sharp
Time:	5–15 seconds

   D. Pattern #3: Swirling

   Choose the point of pain and swirl around it, spiraling outward from the pain.

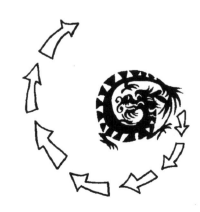

Swirling can also be accomplished, and is most effective in chronic pain, when I start the spiral away from the site of pain and move in the swirling pattern inward to the point.

Hz: 20 Hz
Microamps: 100 µA
Wave Slope: Moderate to Sharp
Time: 5–15 seconds

E. Pattern #5: T.E.S.T. and ETR

Use the hand-held electrode directly opposite the treatment "Q" probe (such as placing the large electrode behind the knee and then treating through the knee with Shotgun, Swirling, or Surrounding procedures).
This is also effective when treating the ankle, foot, hand, shoulder, wrist, or elbow.

Hz: 3–9 Hz
Microamps: 40–100 µA
Wave Slope: Gentle to Moderate
Time: 5–15 seconds

F. Pattern #6: Sequential Treatment

Primarily used for treatment of extremities.
Use when treating acupuncture points on the extremities, starting at the site of pain and moving towards the periphery. Example: for shoulder pain, begin at LI 15 and move to LI 14, 11, etc..

Hz: 4–7 Hz
Microamps: Tolerance
Wave Slope: Sharp
Time: Maximum response

3. One rubber pad and one treatment probe

The pad acts as the indifferent electrode. Place rubber pad on tender point corresponding with site to be treated. Using treatment probe, treat in basic patterns as for single probe. The size of the pad determines the amount of treatment affected at each site of contact. The larger the surface area of the pad, the more diffused the current at that site. The smaller the pad, the more equal the treatment. The closer the pad comes to being the same size as the treatment probe, the more uniform the treatment at each site. You can also use two "Q" probes to provide very specific treatment. Use these principles with any pattern which uses a single treatment probe.

Example: for a shoulder problem, place pad on tender point on neck or back--C5 or T2. Then Shotgun with the treatment "Q" probe.

Instrument settings: Determine according to patterns chosen from Section 2: hand-held electrode and treatment probe

4. Two treatment probes

Used for ETR, EMR, multiple point treatments, concentrated auricular treatments, Golgi tendon and spindle cell procedures, and transcutaneous stimulation.

A. Patterns

1) Use the same patterns as with the single probe, only enhance the effect by placing probes opposite each other or side by side when treating surface areas, or on opposite surfaces when treating through organ areas or through body and joint areas.

2) One probe may be used as a stationary probe on the point of pain. Swirl with the other probe.

3) With one probe stationary at the point of pain, treat each acupoint sequentially with the other probe.

Hz: 20 Hz
Microamps: 100 μA
Wave Slope: Moderate to Sharp
Time: 5–15 seconds

B. Multiple acupuncture points

1) Treat two acupoints simultaneously

2) Treat a primary acupoint with a stationary probe. Treat secondary points with other probe.

Hz: 10 Hz for extremities
                 20 Hz for body
Microamps: 20 μA to patient's tolerance
Wave Slope: Moderate to Sharp
Time: 10–15 seconds

C. Enhancing Tissue Repair (Wing's ETR)

Place affected area between two probes and treat with one of the above patterns (effective in muscle strains, contusions, burns, arthritis of joints, tendonitis, bursitis, sinusitis, infected or weak organs).

Hz: .9 Hz
Microamps: 20–50 μA
Wave Slope: Low to Moderate
Time: 15 seconds

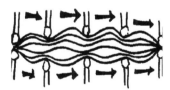

D. Enhancing Muscle Reeducation (Wing's EMR)
   Effective with muscular injury and weakness.

Delineate the muscle and place probes perpendicular to the direction of the muscle fibers. Treat the length of the muscle, starting at the origin and moving towards the insertion, lifting the muscle so as to include as many fibers as possible. Make several passes along the muscle in this manner.

Hz: .1 Hz
Microamps: 50–100 μA   origin
Wave Slope: Moderate
Time: 5–15 seconds   insertion

E. Transcutaneous Electro-Stimulation, Tsunami (Wing's T.E.S.T.)

Place an area of pain between probes. Treat in a similar manner as ETR, except T.E.S.T. can also be used effectively through joints, especially paravertebrally.

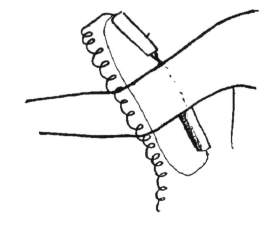

Hz: .3–.9 Hz
Microamps: 40–100 μA
Wave Slope: Gentle to Moderate
Time: 15 seconds

F. Goodheart/Wing Golgi Tendon Procedures

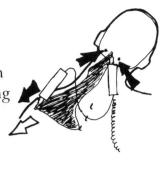

For muscles weakened by injury, place the affected muscle in a stretched position. Treat the hypertonic muscle by stroking towards the origin and insertion, or by treating the Spindle Cells (located in the belly of the muscle) with inward stroking.

Hz formula: .1 Hz x muscle length in inches = Hz setting
Microamps: 40–100 μA
Wave Slope: Gentle to Moderate
Time: Stroking at muscle attachments
or spindle cells, 20 seconds,
repeating as necessary

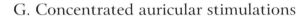

G. Concentrated auricular stimulations

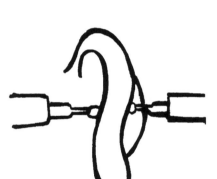

Place treatment probe on appropriate auricular point. Place second probe on back side of ear, as close as possible to a position directly opposite the treatment probe.

Hz formula: 20 Hz or variable Hz if using
Nogier's procedures
Microamps: To tolerance
Wave Slope: Moderate
Time: 10 sec. to maximum response

H. Simultaneous stimulation

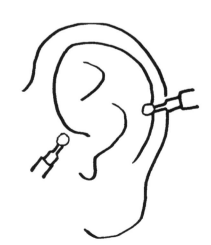

Choose which auricular points should be treated, and treat them two at a time (example: Point Zero and Shoulder, or Allergy and Adrenal).

Hz formula: 20 Hz or variable Hz if using
Nogier's procedures
Microamps: To tolerance
Wave Slope: Moderate
Time: 10 sec. to maximum response

5. Double Pads

    A. Place one pad on tender point along spine and the other on the site of pain.
    B. Put the site of pain between two pads.

    For an enkephalin response (relief while current is on)
    Hz: 8 Hz
    Microamps: To tolerance
    Wave Slope: Gentle
    Time: 10–30 minutes

    For endorphin response
    Hz: 3 to 10 Hz
    Microamps: To tolerance
    Wave Slope: Sharp
    Time: 5–15 seconds or
                     maximum response

    For reduction of swelling--used   mostly on sprains
    and on real acutes

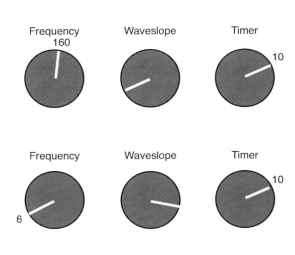

    Hz: 300 Hz
    Microamps: Patient's tolerance
    Wave Slope: Gentle
    Time: 10 minutes

    then change to
    Hz: 160 Hz
    Microamps: Patient's tolerance
    Wave Slope: Gentle
    Time: 10 minutes

    then change to
    Hz: 6 Hz
    Microamps: Patient's tolerance
    Wave Slope: Sharp
    Time: 10 minutes

To accelerate healing, use for a longer period of treatment time. To reduce
swelling, double or triple the time on 300 and 160 Hz settings according to
degree of injury.   Treat at 6 Hz for 10 minutes. On sprains, follow up working
on the muscle using ETR, EMR, T.E.S.T., etc..

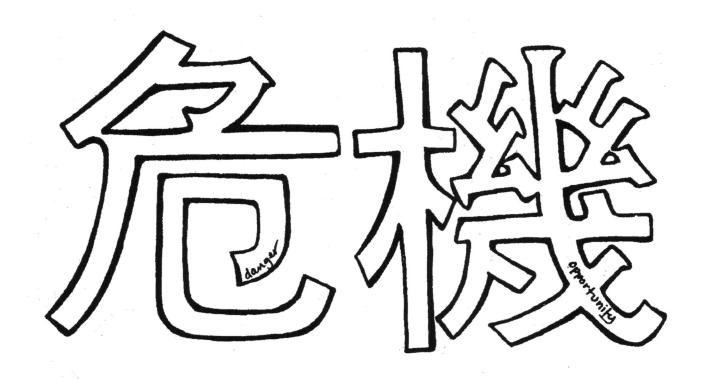

"crisis"

EAR-RICULAR THERAPY

EAR-RICULAR THERAPY
Auricular Therapy According To Wing

On the ear, as on the iris, the hand, and the bottom of the foot, is a map of the body. Dr. Thomas W. Wing organized the ear points into groups, linking them together like constellations of stars. On his chart, they are connected by lines. By using ear landmarks, you will be able to find all the points in the group, tracing out the pattern. For example, you can locate A6 by looking at the bottom near the level of the Concha and then tracing backwards to the end of the line.

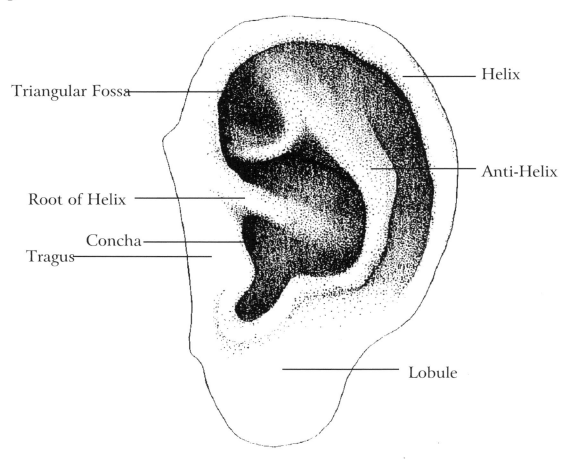

PARTS OF THE EAR

SEE-DO EAR-RICULAR POINTS

A GROUP: arm

A1 fingers
A2 wrist
A3 elbow
A4 shoulder
A5 shoulder joint
A6 clavicle

B GROUP: lower extremities

B1   toes
B2   heel
B3   ankle
B4   knee
B5   hip
B6   hip joint
B7   buttock
B8   abdomen
B9   chest
B9A   mammary gland
B9B   mammary gland
B10   neck
B11   upper neck
B10A thyroid 2

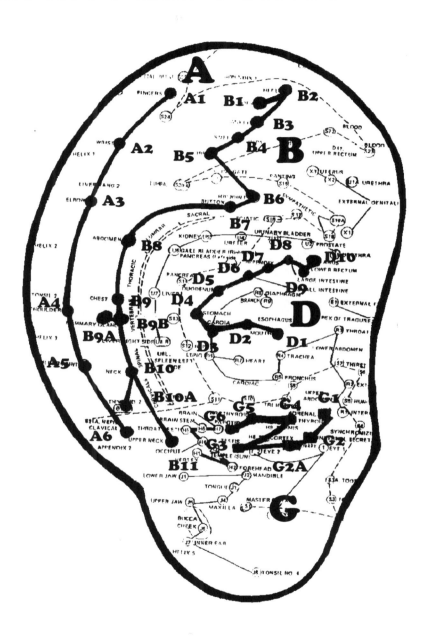

A GROUP: arm

D1	mouth	D6	small intestine
D2	esophagus	D7	appendix
D3	cardia	D8	large intestine
D4	stomach	D9	lower rectum
D5	duodenum	D10	anus

G GROUP: glands

G1	adrenal		
G2	internal secretions		
G2A	ovary		
G3	testis	G5	parathyroid
G4	thyroid	G6	parotid

43

E GROUP: ear

E1   external ear
E2   apex of tragus

I GROUP: eye

I   eye
I-2 eye 1
I-3 eye 2

J GROUP: jaw

J1   lower jaw
J2   mandible
J3   tongue
J4   maxilla
J5   upper jaw
J6   bucca cheek
J7   inner ear
J8   tonsil 4

S GROUP:
symptoms

S1   Master of Pain
S2   Nerve pain (yin)
S3   Tooth pain
S3A   Tooth (yang)
S4   Synchronizing Point
S5   Hunger
S6   Mute Gate
S7   Thirst
S8   Cardiac (yang)
S9   Tri Heater
S10   Lung (yin)
S11   Tooth (yang)
S11A   Kidney (yang)
S12   Liver (yin)
S13   Liver (yang)
S14   Pancreas (yang)
S15   Fluid (yin)
S16   Sciatic nerve (yang)
S17   Colon (yang)
S18   Sympathetic #1
S18A   Sympathetic #2

S19   Panting
S20   Divine Gate
S21   Liver (yang)
S22   Blood (yin)
S23   Blood (yang)
S24   Skin (yang)
S25   Minor Occipital Nerve
S26   Allergy

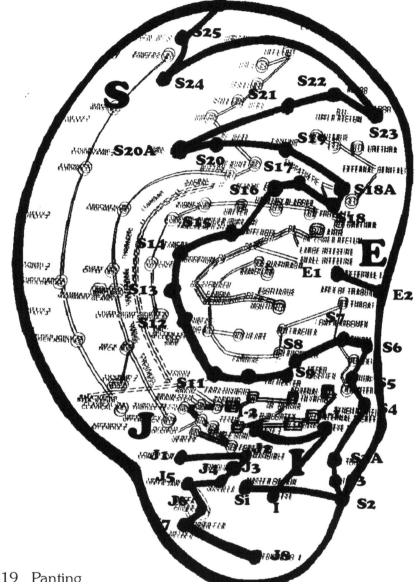

H GROUP: head

H1 Vertex
H2 Forehead
H3 Temple (sun)
H4 Occiput
H5 Throat Teeth
H6 Brain Stem
H7 Brain
H8 Subcortex
H9 Dermis

R GROUP: respiratory

R1 Internal nose
R2 External nose
R3 Throat
R4 Trachea
R5 Bronchus
R6 Lung
R7 Heart
R8 Diaphragm
R9 Branch

U GROUP: urinary

U1 Urethra
U2 Prostate
U3 Urinary bladder
U4 Ureter
U5 Kidney
U6 Gallbladder (R)
U6 Pancreas (L)
U7 Liver
U8 Liver (R)
U8 Spleen (L)

X GROUP: sex

X1 External genitalia
X2 External genitalia
X3 Uterus

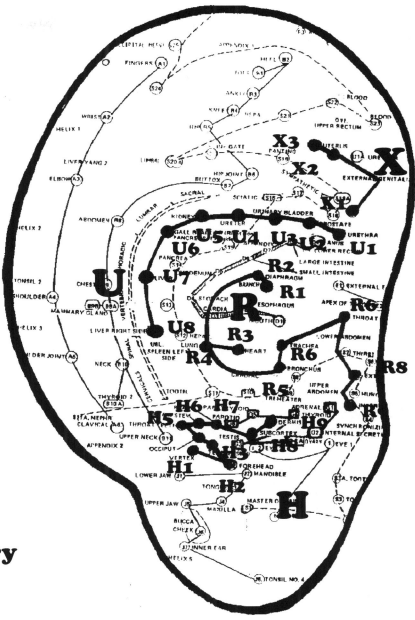

EAR SCAN

The ear is like a computer terminal of the body. There are more than a hundred acu-points on it. These indicate, by change in electrical conductance, whenever changes occur in the body. You can chart these imbalances with a small-tipped metal probe. Some people like the stainless steel curved auricular probe, but it has a very small tip and the practitioner must use extreme caution to avoid scratching the ear. Dr. Greenlee prefers the brass probes because they are more sensitive to electrical conductance. If you use a brass probe, you must also use a brass hand mass. The "Q" probe has too large a tip to give accurate readings on an ear scan. However, many practitioners prefer the "Q" for treating because it does not sting the patient. What about the hazard of treating points that are near the points chosen for treatment? Those who use "Q" probes for treating believe acupoints which require treatment will accept the current and those that don't won't.

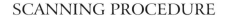

SCANNING PROCEDURE

1. Scan the ear by drawing the tip of probe along the groove of the Helix, starting with point A1 (fingers). If readings are too low, try turning the sensitivity knob (if you have one) up higher.

2. With a tape recorder or the help of an assistant, record the reading from the meter.

3. Sometimes the patient feels pain; acupoints which are way out of balance do hurt sometimes. Pain with a high reading is a very yang imbalance. Pain with a very low reading or no reading at all is a very yin imbalance. Be sure to note pain readings on your chart. We put a little "x" by the number.

4. Search whichever groups you desire. No variation in readings and no pain means no imbalance. Points will be less sore, respond more quickly, and be fewer as the patient gains internal balance.

   You will find that ear points on charts vary. That is because people are individuals and their points don't always match the model. Also, points may change as conditions change. Dr. Nogier discovered that points change with the progression of a condition.

REFERRED PAIN EAR-RICULAR TESTS

Sometimes pain or restriction of motion is referred from another area. The following chart describes the tests which indicate problems coming from specific meridians. To use these tests, have your patient move according to the tests described below. When you find restriction or pain, treat the ear-ricular point corresponding to the meridian indicated at 20 Hz for 10 seconds at 40 μA. If the pain or restriction changes for the better, further investigation is warranted.

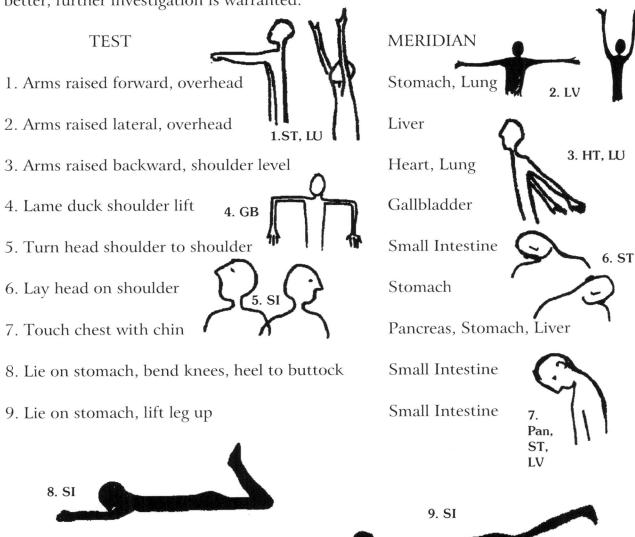

TEST	MERIDIAN
1. Arms raised forward, overhead	Stomach, Lung
2. Arms raised lateral, overhead	Liver
3. Arms raised backward, shoulder level	Heart, Lung
4. Lame duck shoulder lift	Gallbladder
5. Turn head shoulder to shoulder	Small Intestine
6. Lay head on shoulder	Stomach
7. Touch chest with chin	Pancreas, Stomach, Liver
8. Lie on stomach, bend knees, heel to buttock	Small Intestine
9. Lie on stomach, lift leg up	Small Intestine

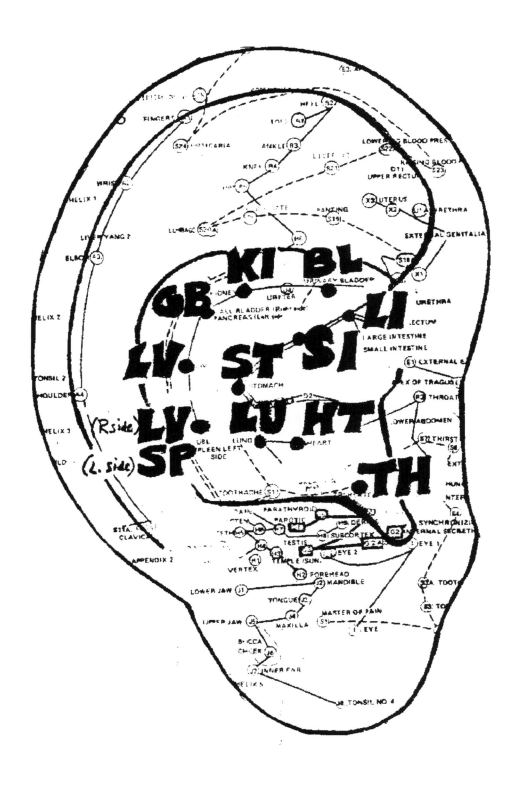

EAR MERIDIAN POINTS

EAR-RICULAR TREATMENT PROCEDURE

1. Inquire about your patient's discomfort, limitations in range of motion, etc.

2. Select the appropriate points for treatment.

3. Set up the instrument.

    A. Set Audible Search Threshold completely to the left, unless you're doing Nogier's work.
    B. Turn Volume to a comfortable level.
    C. If you are using a metal probe, set Frequency to lowest microamps. For "Q" probe, set it for mid-range up to 100 μA— best at lowest level.
    D. Prepare Q-tip and insert, or insert ball tip or auricular probe.
    E. Set timer to 5–10 seconds.
    F. Set GSR (Galvanic Skin Resistance control if you have it) to measure sensitivity or High resistance.

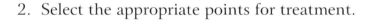

Threshold

Volume

Current

4. Place indifferent electrode in the hand of the patient.

5. With instrument on Search, place probe firmly on the site to be treated at approximately a 90° angle.

6. Support the back of the ear if you're treating points on the front, or pull the ear back with the other hand to expose points on the rear of the ear.

NOTE: Do not allow the metal shaft of the probe to touch anywhere else on the patient or you. The only contact with the patient should be probe tip and your supporting hand.

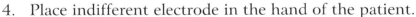
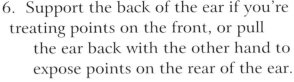
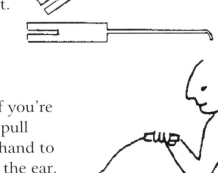
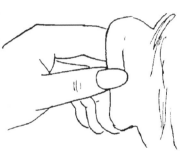
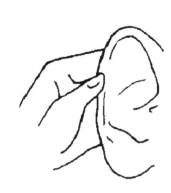

8. Press the button on the handle while maintaining contact with the probe. Do not move the probe until after the treatment cycle has finished.

9. Evaluate acupoint response.

10. Remove probe from acupoint. Treat the other points selected in the same way.

11. Ask the patient to reevaluate the condition or area of complaint.

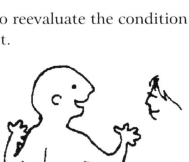

SEQUENTIAL TREATMENTS

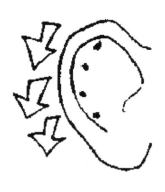

yang

It is possible to give sequential treatments in the ear—both to move energy into an area, and to move it out. If your patient has pains in the shoulder, treat Group A in a yin direction (from the shoulder to the fingers). If he has numbness in his fingers, treat in a yang direction. Each stimulation should be given to maximum response. Use the frequency which you find the most effective. Dr. Wing uses 2.5 Hz. Robert Peshek, D.D.S., uses 20 Hz. James Greenlee, D.C., uses 10 Hz.

yin

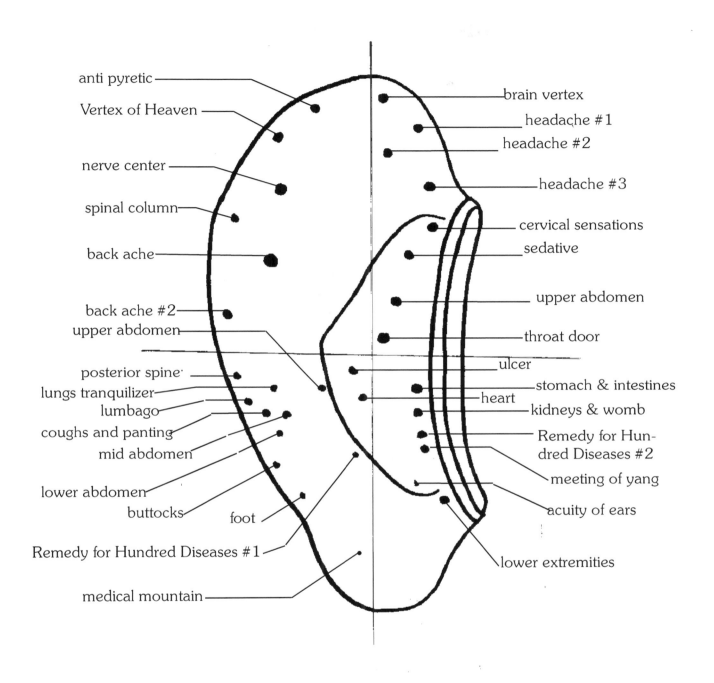

anti pyretic

Vertex of Heaven

nerve center

spinal column

back ache

back ache #2

upper abdomen

posterior spine

lungs tranquilizer

lumbago

coughs and panting

mid abdomen

lower abdomen

buttocks

foot

Remedy for Hundred Diseases #1

medical mountain

brain vertex

headache #1

headache #2

headache #3

cervical sensations

sedative

upper abdomen

throat door

ulcer

stomach & intestines

heart

kidneys & womb

Remedy for Hundred Diseases #2

meeting of yang

acuity of ears

lower extremities

THE REAR OF THE EAR

51

SPECIAL FEATURES OF THE EAR
Dennis L. Greenlee, D.C., L.Ac.

The ear has special significance in the treatment of pain as well as for organic therapy. The external ear develops from the embryonic gill plates. This is the only structure whose tissue develops from the three embryonic layers of the body: ectoderm, mesoderm, and endoderm. The ectodermal segment is the helix and lobe of the ear, while the mesodermal segment is the pinna, and the endodermal segment is the concha. The contact reflexes are located in those specific developmental layers within the ear. As disease progresses, it passes through those germ layers.

The ear is also an important area for contact reflex treatment because of its neurological innervation. The helix and lobe are innervated by the greater auricular nerve of the superior cervical plexus (C1-C2-C3). The Pinna is innervated by the anterior superior branch of the trigeminal nerve (Cranial V). The concha and tragus innervation is from the vagus (Cranial X), trigeminal (Cranial V) and facial (Cranial VII) and the glossopharyngeal (Cranial IX). The significance of innervation is the convergence of its spinothalamic and cerebrospinal fibers within the reticular area in the spinal cord and brain stem. Because of this connection, their afferent fibers descend and have a direct effect on the periphery of the body.

One of the greatest benefits comes from the ear's ability to affect the parasympathetic influence to organs and vascular system as well as its ability to affect the central nervous system. It is the only external contact to the vagus nerve. The ear acts as transmitter-receiver which is in direct contact with the central nervous system.

The Progression of Conditions

It has been discovered that ear points and the associated tissues correspond to the embryonic developments of those tissues.

The **Mesodermal** tissues include the musculoskeletal tissues and, from an auricular viewpoint, the dermis and adrenals, kidneys, and ureter.

Endodermal tissue development reflects all other organs of the abdomen and chest, including the thyroid and parathyroid.

The **Ectodermal** relationship includes the spinal cord, brain, and the glands within the skull.

The Progression of Conditions reprinted from *The Healing Ear, Intermediate Auricular Therapy* p.6 by Dennis L. Greenlee, D.C., L.Ac. published by Earthen Vessel Productions, 1995. Used by permission.

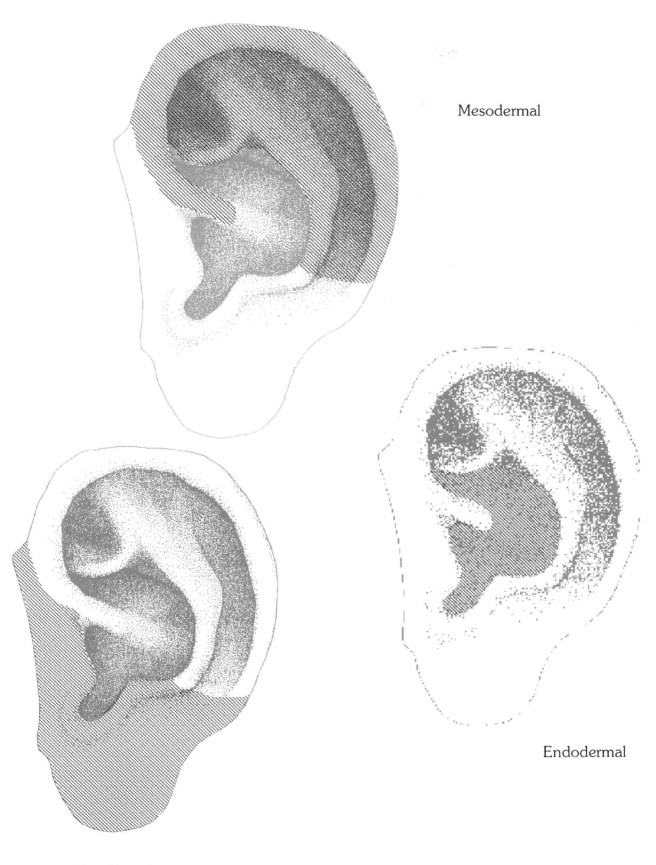

Mesodermal

Endodermal

Ectodermal

53

Master Control Points

The Master Control Points of the ear are used to open systems before treatment. They can also be used for general tonification. Choose points according to function and treat for 15 to 20 seconds per point.

Point Zero - 10 Hz
> ~ Brings the body into a general balance
> ~ Facilitates willpower

Shen Men - 10 Hz
> ~ Alleviates pain, tension, and anxiety
> ~ Quiets the mind and heart

Sympathetic Tone - 10 Hz
> ~ Balances the activities of the sympathetic nervous system
> ~ Improves vascular tone

Thalamus Point - 80 Hz
> ~ Reduces pain by its effect on the gate control pathways

Endocrine Hormones Point – 80 Hz
> ~ Balances endocrine system by raising or lowering
>   the secretions of the pituitary

Oscillation Point - 2.5 Hz
> ~ Balances right and left cerebral hemispheres
> ~ Corrects cerebral laterality

Stress Control Point - 20 Hz
> ~ Activates ACTH and corticosteroid hormones

Tranquilizer Point - 20 Hz
> ~ Used for high blood pressure
> ~ Relaxes the body and mind
> ~ Is a Valium analogue point

Master Sensorial Point - 160 Hz
> ~ Reduces unpleasant or excessive sensations

Master Cerebral Point - 160 Hz
> ~ Reduces fear, worry, nervousness
> ~ Produces analgesia
> ~ Psychosomatic point

Master Control Points of the Ear reprinted from *The Healing Ear, Intermediate Auricular Therapy* pages 22 & 23 by Dennis L. Greenlee, D.C., L.Ac. published by Earthen Vessel Productions, 1995. Used by permission.

Master Control Points

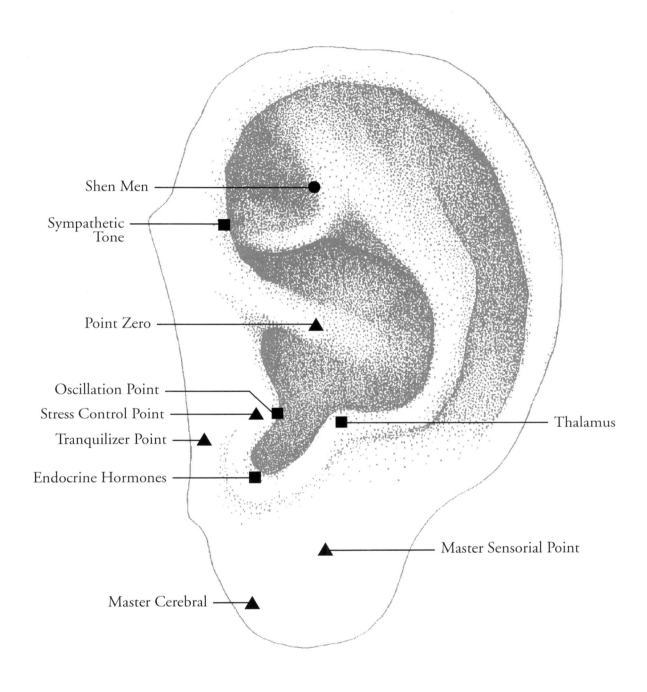

Shen Men

Sympathetic Tone

Point Zero

Oscillation Point

Stress Control Point

Tranquilizer Point

Endocrine Hormones

Thalamus

Master Sensorial Point

Master Cerebral

● Depressed

■ Wall

▲ Elevated

Greenlee Meridian Balance Chart

Name_____ Date_____ Time_____ a.m./p.m.

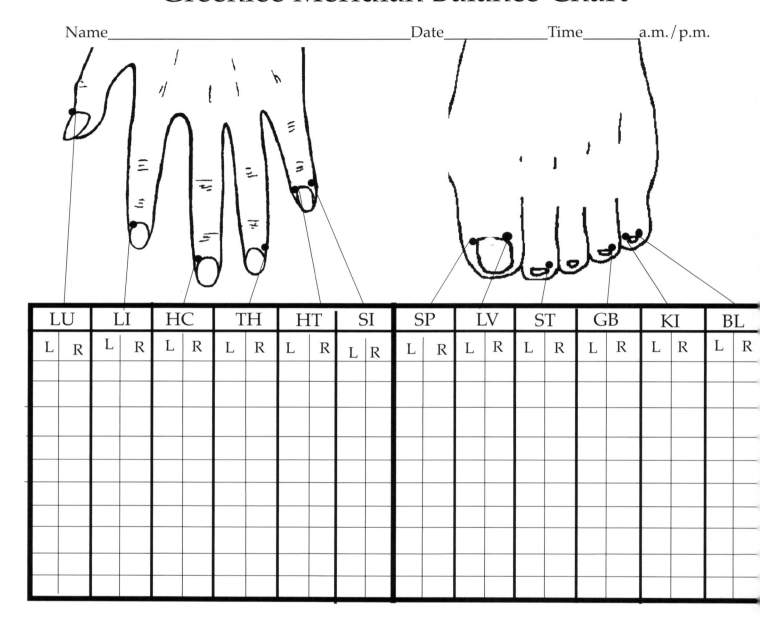

LU		LI		HC		TH		HT		SI		SP		LV		ST		GB		KI		BL	
L	R	L	R	L	R	L	R	L	R	L	R	L	R	L	R	L	R	L	R	L	R	L	R

MERIDIAN THERAPY

MERIDIANS

For the Western mind, often one of the most troublesome aspects of Chinese medicine is the concept of meridians—the invisible lines of energy in the body which seem as imaginary as dragons and monkey gods. In more recent times, however, western researchers have investigated these lines and discovered that they were electronically traceable. They found the charts of the ancients to be astoundingly accurate—even to the loop of the Kidney meridian on the ankle.

Though energetic medicine is not so foreign to some groups of health professionals, there are still concepts and terms which may be unfamiliar. This section contains brief explanations of the basic terms.

MERIDIANS: Meridians are channels of energy which run in very specific pathways throughout the body. There are twelve major meridians—each named for the major organ which most greatly influences it. Following the order of testing with Akabane Points, they are: Lung, Large Intestine, Tri Heater (or Triple Warmer), Heart Constrictor (or Pericardium), Heart, Small Intestine, Spleen, Liver, Gallbladder, Stomach, Kidney, and Bladder.

There are two meridian names which do not represent organs, but functions. These are Heart Constrictor and Tri Heater. The Heart Constrictor deals primarily with circulation. The Tri Heater deals primarily with lymphatic distribution and the endocrine system.

Two other vessels are the Conception Vessel and the Governing Vessel. They are not bilateral. The Conception Vessel ("CV" or "VC") runs up the front of the body. The Governing Vessel ("GV") runs up the back. Both vessels connect to all energetic systems, nourish all internal organs and viscera, and govern many physiological functions.

In their flow patterns, the twelve meridians are bilateral, although, for clarity in the illustrations which follow this section, the meridians are shown only on one side of the body. The dotted lines represent the deep flow and show the relationship to the organs of the body.

FUNCTIONS OF MERIDIANS

LUNG	Diseases of lungs, chest, throat, and upper extremities
PERICARDIUM	Diseases of chest, heart, stomach, and upper extremities
HEART	Diseases of chest, heart and upper extremities
LARGE INTESTINE	Diseases of large intestine, head, face, eyes, nose, mouth, teeth, throat, and upper extremities
TRI HEATER	Lateral side of head, eyes, ears, throat, and upper extremities
SMALL INTESTINE	Diseases of small intestine, head, neck, eyes, ears, throat, and upper extremities
SPLEEN	Diseases of spleen, pancreas, abdomen, urogenital system, stomach, intestines, and lower extremities
LIVER	Diseases of liver, abdomen, urogenital system, and joints and ligaments
KIDNEY	Diseases of kidney, lung, throat, abdomen, urogenital areas, intestines, and lower extremities
STOMACH	Diseases of stomach, head, face, mouth, teeth, throat, intestines, and lower extremities
GALLBLADDER	Diseases of gall bladder, lateral aspect of head, eyes, ears, costal and subcostal region, and lower extremities
BLADDER	Diseases of bladder, head, neck, eyes, back, lower extremities, and gluteal region

In the international designation of acupoints, points are numbered, each starting with the number 1. You can tell which way the energy flows by starting with the first point and following the pathway as the numbers increase. Bladder 67 is on the little toe. Bladder 1 is in the head. Therefore, the Bladder meridian travels from the head to the foot. Each meridian has one end (either the first or the last point in the series) located on either a finger or a toe.

MERIDIAN FLOW

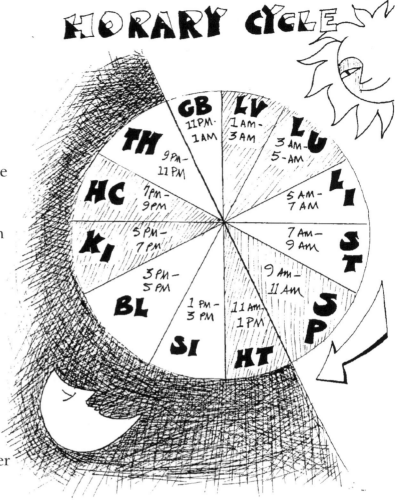

Meridians are not a closed system of individual paths; they are connected to each other. One of the five energetic exchanges among the twelve principal bilateral channels is called the Circadian or Horary Cycle. Energy flows through them in a specific order as follows:

Lung to Large Intestine
Large Intestine to Stomach
Stomach to Spleen
Spleen to Heart
Heart to Small Intestine
Small Intestine to Bladder
Bladder to Kidney
Kidney to Heart Constrictor
Heart Constrictor to Tri Heater
Tri Heater to Gallbladder
Gallbladder to Liver
Liver to Lung

According to the ancient Chinese theory, each meridian has two hours during which it is at its maximum and two hours during which its energy is at its minimum. If a patient has a reoccurring problem at a specific time, checking the Horary Cycle chart may give you a clue as to where that problem really lies.

If an organ is stimulated moderately, only the organ itself is affected (strengthened), but strong stimulation creates a sedation effect in the organ opposite the one being treated (example: GB stimulated too long would cause sedation in HT).

If an organ is weak, it can benefit greatly from being stimulated at its peak time (a granule can be attached to the acupoint involved and the patient instructed to press on it at the appropriate time). In more crucial cases, a home stimulator such as the Freedom Micro can be helpful for self-treatment.

COUPLED MERIDIANS: Meridians are paired according to their positions on the front and back of the body. Each pair of coupled meridians has one yin and one yang meridian. The yang meridians are on the back of the body. The yin ones are on the front. Since the outsides of things, the surfaces, are yang, one way to visualize this is to picture a baby crawling. His back is the outside. His front is on the yinside.

The Chinese consider the solid organs to be yin and the hollow ones to be yang. This is another way to remember which meridians are which. The bladder is the hollow organ. Its meridian is on the back. The Bladder Meridian is the yang, while the Kidney Meridian, representing the solid organ, is the yin. It is on the front. Yin meridians run up the front of the body and yang ones run down the back or sides. The exception is the Governing Vessel, a yang meridian which runs up the back. Generally, a yin organ is benefitted by stimulation at a yin time (noon to midnight), and a yang organ at a yang time (midnight to noon).

THE LAW OF THE FIVE ELEMENTS

Each of the pairs of meridians is associated with an element. The elements are WOOD, WATER, FIRE, EARTH, and METAL. These associations are both metabolic according to function and, startlingly enough, sometimes observable. A metallic taste in the mouth, for example, often indicates a problem in the Lung.

Wood:	Liver and Gallbladder
Water:	Kidney and Bladder
Fire:	Heart and Small Intestine
Fire:	Tri Heater and Heart Constrictor
Earth:	Spleen and Stomach
Metal:	Lung and Large Intestine

Each of the elements is associated with a sense, a liquid, and has a system it nourishes.

ASPECT:	METAL	FIRE	EARTH	WOOD	WATER
Sense:	smell	words	taste	sight	hearing
Liquid:	mucus	sweat	saliva	tears	urine
Nourishes:	skin	blood vessels	fat	muscles	bone

The elements interact with each other in several exchanges. One of them, the Circadian Cycle, has already been described. The other two are the Generating and Controlling Cycles.

61

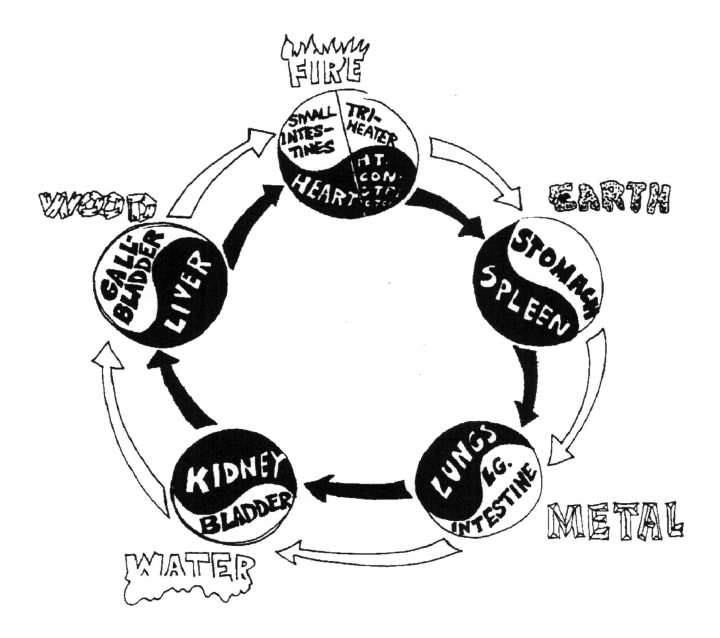

THE GENERATING CYCLE

Perhaps the ancients thought of the Generating Cycle this way:
Water nourishes Wood, Wood feeds Fire, Fire reduces to Earth, Earth creates Metal,
Metal nourishes Water (by adding minerals such as iron).

THE CONTROLLING CYCLE

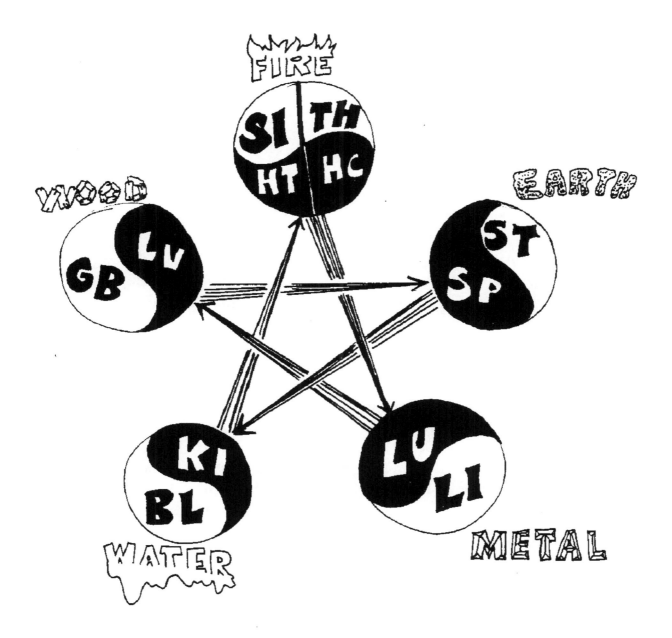

In the Controlling Cycle, Water quenches Fire, Fire melts Metal, Metal chops Wood, Wood devours Earth, Earth absorbs Water.

MERIDIAN THERAPY

Rather than labeling a myriad of diseases, the Chinese identify the relative relationships of energies within the body, recognizing that these relationships are in a state of flux. When a person catches a cold, his symptoms (cold, fever, nasal congestion) are external, that is, yang. As the symptoms internalize (coughing and phlegm), the condition is considered to be more yin. Pneumonia develops as the lungs, exhausted from coughing, lose energy.

The paired yang and yin meridians are coupled by connecting points (also called Luo Points). At these points, where meridian polarity changes take place, we can most easily influence the flow of energy.

PULSE DIAGNOSIS VS ELECTRICAL MEASUREMENTS

Robert Ripley of "Ripley's Believe It or Not" frequently quoted an old Chinese saying: The Chinese hire their physician when they are well, and fire them if they become ill. This is because the meridians can be monitored by pulse diagnosis, and if the physician keeps them in balance, the patient will stay well. Reading the twelve pulses is a very difficult and time consuming technic to master, however. How could the Western world gain the benefits of this ancient art?

A breakthrough occurred when Dr. Yoshio Nakatani of Japan verified the meridian concept in 1950 when he discovered that acupoints could be measured with electrical current. Dr. Nakatani used Source Points located on the wrists, hands, ankles and feet for his measurements. The search probe was either a large cotton swab about 3/8 inch in diameter or a sharp one millimeter metallic one. The larger one was too broad to be very accurate, and the smaller one could cause DC burns. The current altered the readings so the points could not be immediately retested.

In 1973, Dr. Wing developed a simpler system by adapting to electrical measurement the beginning or end points of the meridians on the fingers and toes. Dr. Akabane was the first to experiment with those points, and he did so by noting the patient's sensitivity to the heat of a stick of incense. Dr. Wing used low voltage electrical current which would not significantly alter the readings of the points and was not as upsetting to his patients. Because the Akabane Points were easy to locate and efficient indicators, they lent themselves to automated readout by his instrument. Thus the wonderful world of meridian therapy became accessible and measurable to Western practitioners.

MERIDIAN CHARTS SHOWING DEEP AND SUPERFICIAL FLOW

Meridian measurements are extremely useful in practicing traditional Chinese medicine. Not only do they suggest the balance of the organs, they also monitor changes in stability, the efficacy of therapy, as well as the energy level of the body at the moment.

Meridian measurements are also helpful for those who do not practice traditional Chinese medicine. Persistent pain can sometimes be referred from an organ. For example, a shoulder problem could be caused by a blockage of the Large or Small Intestine meridians. A look at which meridians flow through the area of pain can give the practitioner another avenue of approach for treatment.

There are many readily available detailed charts of the meridians. The charts which follow are simplified; there are no letters or numbers. Meridians are bilateral (except for the Conception and Governing Vessels), but these charts show only one side to make it look less confusing. The solid lines show the superficial flow of energy; dotted lines indicate the deep flow. These charts are not meant to be perfect meridian charts. They are provided simply to give you an idea of the flow of each individual meridian as it runs through the body. The order of their appearance in the following pages matches the order that they occur on the fingers and toes in Akabane Testing (see p. 80). At the bottom of each chart is a list of diseases associated with that meridian and its weak and strong times according to the Horary Cycle (see p. 60).

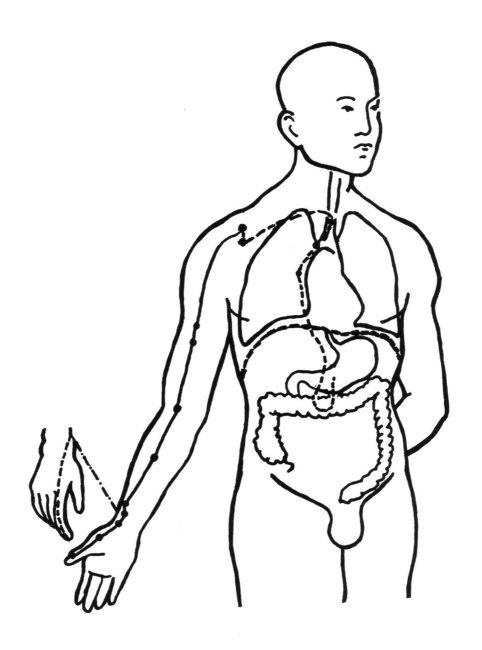

LUNG MERIDIAN

diseases of chest, lungs, throat, and upper extremities
febrile diseases
strong 3 A.M–5 A.M., weak 3 P.M–5 P.M.

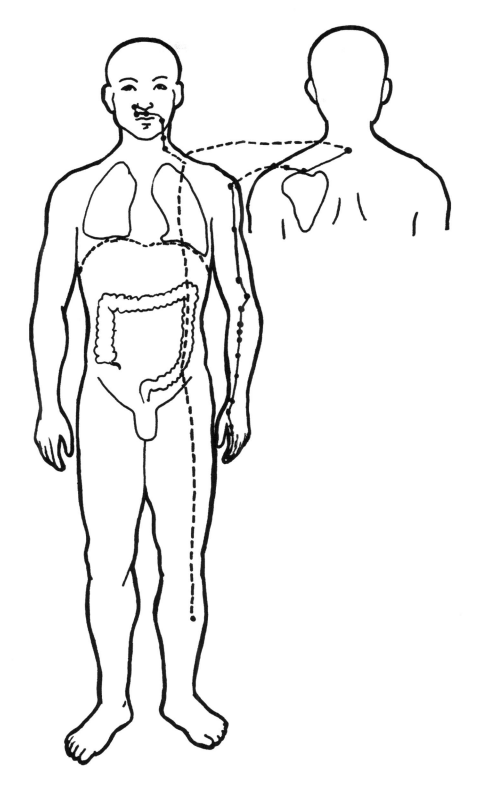

LARGE INTESTINE

diseases of head, face, eyes, nose, mouth, teeth, throat, and upper extremities
febrile diseases
strong 5 A.M.–7 A.M., weak 5 P.M.–7 P.M.

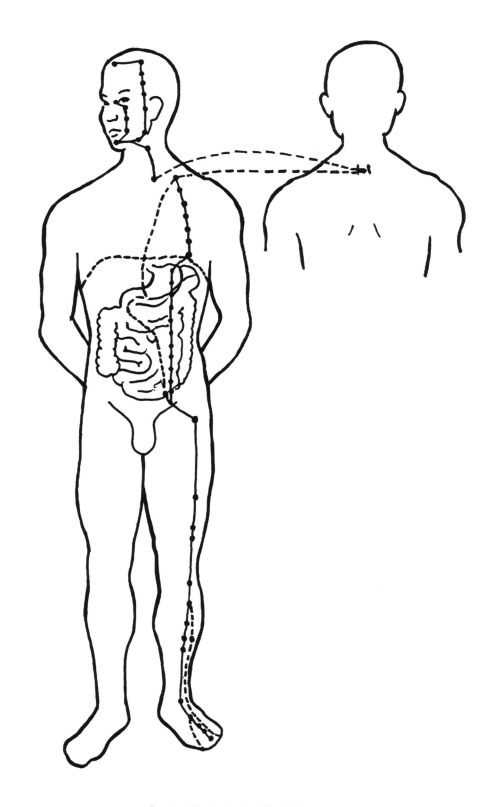

STOMACH

Diseases of head, face, mouth, teeth, throat, stomach, intestines, and lower extremities
febrile diseases, disturbed sensorium
strong 7A.M.–9 A.M., weak 7 P.M.–9 P.M.

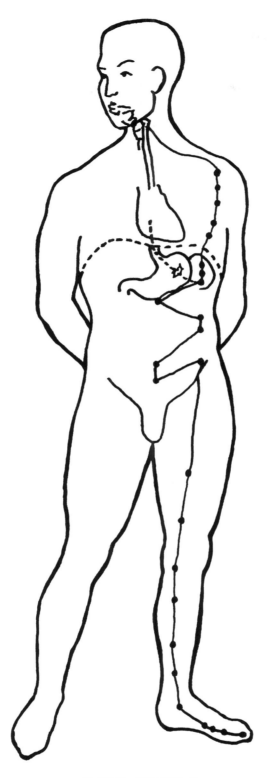

SPLEEN

diseases of abdomen, urogenital system, stomach, intestines and lower extremities
diseases of the cold syndrome
strong 9 A.M.–11 A.M., weak 9 P.M.–11 P.M.

69

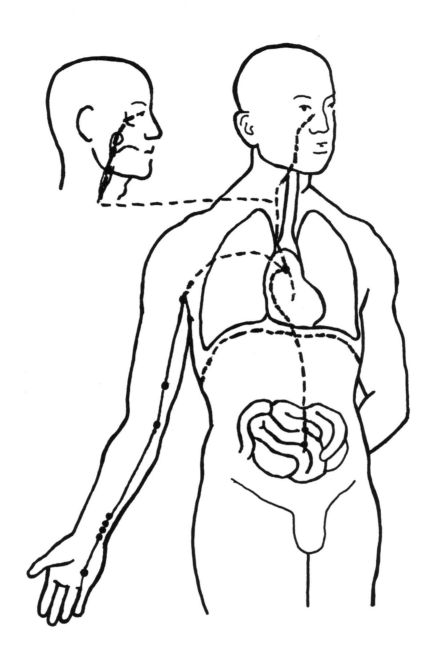

HEART

diseases of chest, heart, and upper extremities
disturbed sensorium
strong 11 A.M.–1 P.M., weak 11 P.M.–1 A.M.

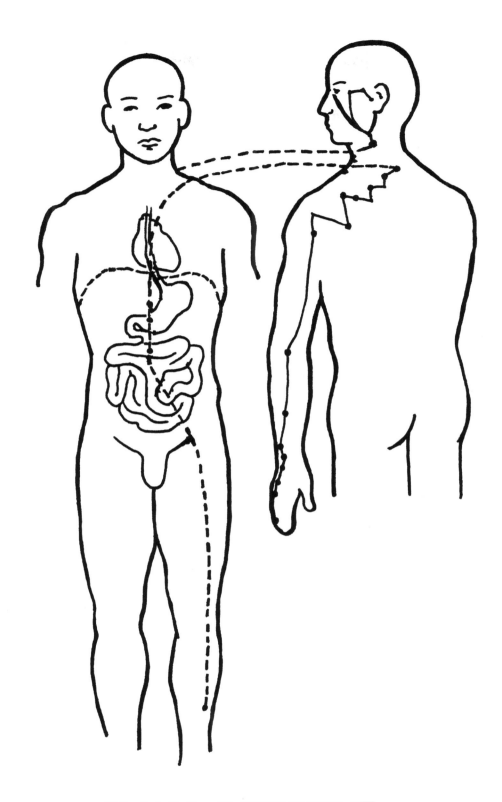

SMALL INTESTINE

diseases of head, neck, eyes, ears, throat, and upper extremities
febrile and mental disorders
strong 1 P.M.–3 P.M., weak 1 A.M.–3 A.M.

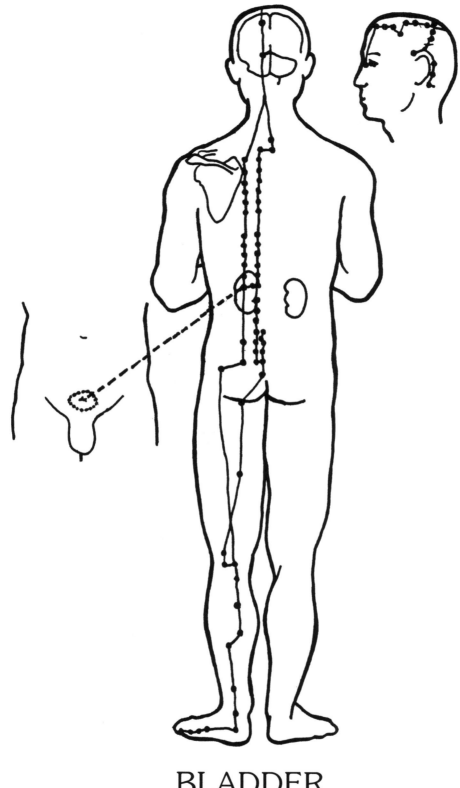

BLADDER

diseases of head, neck, eyes, back, lower extremities, and gluteal region
febrile and mental disorders
strong 3 P.M.–5 P.M., weak 3 A.M.–5 A.M.

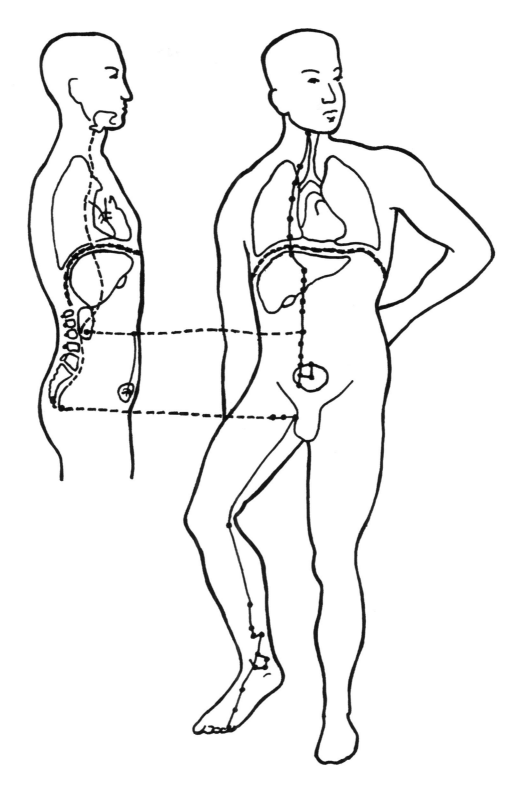

KIDNEY

diseases of lung, throat, abdominal and urogenital regions, intestinal tract, and lower extremities
febrile diseases
strong 5 P.M.–7 P.M., weak 5 A.M.–7 A.M.

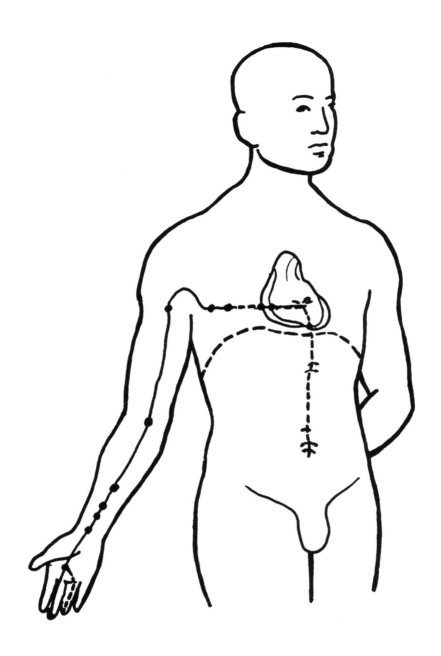

HEART CONSTRICTOR
(Pericardium)
diseases of chest, heart, stomach, and upper extremities
disturbed sensorium
strong 7 P.M.–9 P.M., weak 7 A.M.–9 A.M.

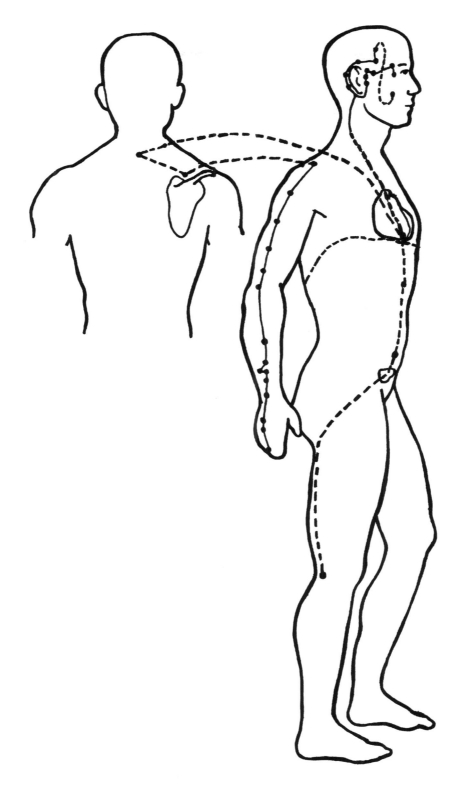

TRI-HEATER • (Triple Warmer)
lateral side of head, eyes, ears, throat, and upper extremities
febrile and mental disorders
strong 9 P.M.–11 P.M., weak 9 A.M.–11 A.M.

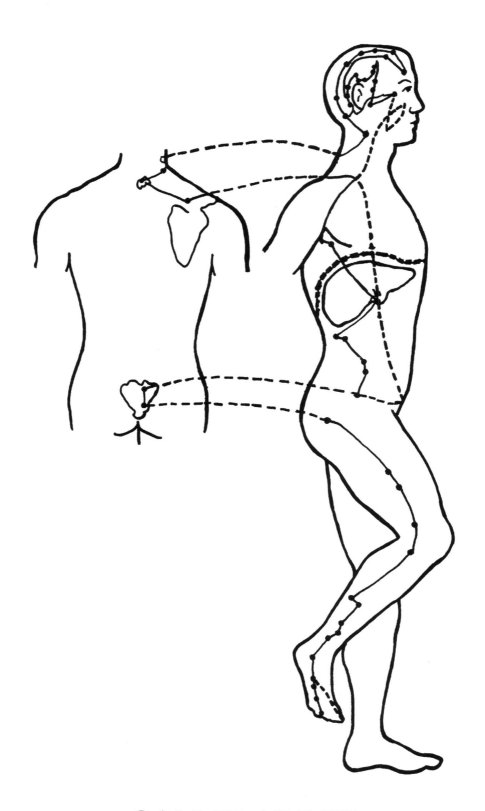

GALLBLADDER

diseases of lateral aspect of head, eyes, ears, costal and subcostal region, and lower extremities
febrile diseases
strong 11 P.M.–1 A.M., weak 11 A.M.–1 P.M.

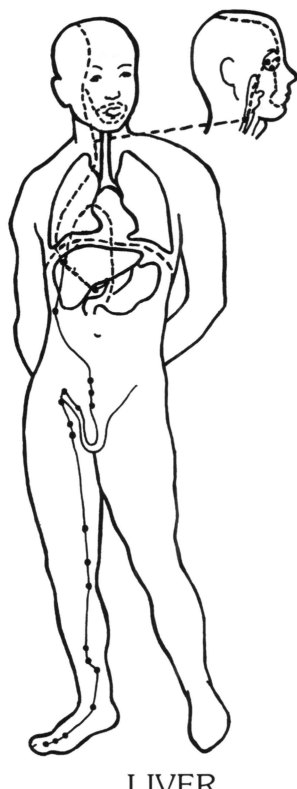

LIVER

diseases of metabolism, abdomen, urogenital system, and joints and ligaments
mental disorders
strong 1 A.M.–3 A.M., weak 1 P.M.–3 P.M.

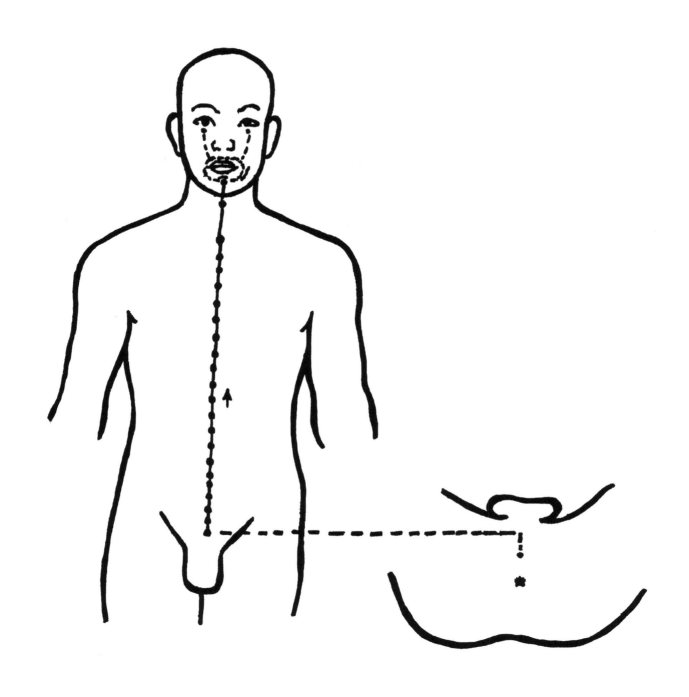

CONCEPTION VESSEL

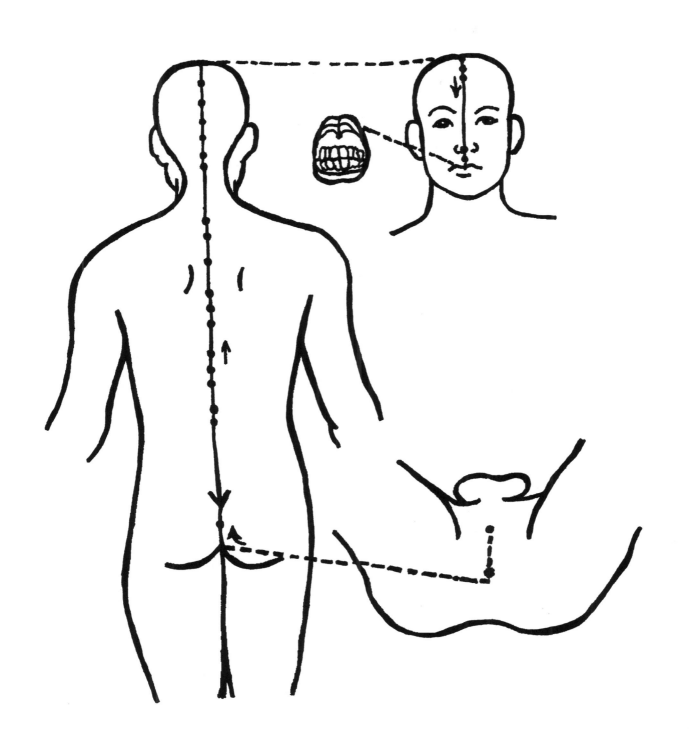

GOVERNING VESSEL

AKABANE/WING
MERIDIAN BALANCE TESTING

One of the most effective ways of determining where energy is blocked and what kind of imbalance (yin or yang) it is manifesting is through a meridian balance chart. We measure the electrical resistance of the points located on the fingers and toes. Since Dr. Akabane was the first to use them for energy testing, we call them Akabane Points. They are located at the intersections of the side of the nail and the cuticle.

Watch for rashes, cuts, abrasions, or cuticles which will give high readings. Calluses give very low readings. If you have a very low reading on the Heart Constrictor, you may be reading a callous. On the Bladder point, you might be reading a corn. Move to the next point along the meridian and take your reading there. It is also important to use consistent pressure. The harder you push, the higher to reading (up to a point, of course). Use firm pressure of about the same amount as needed to write with a ball point pen. Do not squeeze the acupoint. This can change the reading.

TAKING READINGS

1. Ask the patient to remove his or her shoes to allow the skin to adjust to room temperature. Excess heat can cause higher readings than are actually indicative of your patient's condition.

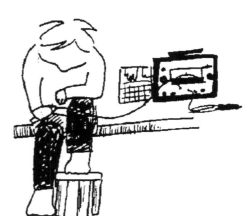

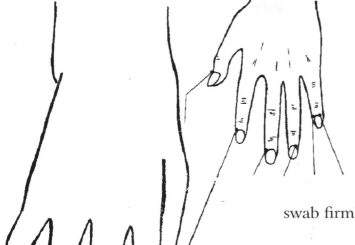

2   Place the indifferent electrode firmly in the hand of the patient, contralateral to the side being tested.

3   Locate the Akabane Point according to the chart. Using the "Q" single probe electrode holder, apply the wetted cotton swab firmly to the chosen point.

4. The pitch and meter reading will rise when the probe contacts the skin. After allowing about one second for the readings to stabilize, record the reading on the chart. To help facilitate interpretation of the chart, record the readings from the right side of the body in red ink, and those from the left in black or blue.

5. Check all the fingers of one hand and all the toes of the foot on the same side. Then change pen colors and check all the fingers and toes of the other side. (You can do both hands and then both feet, but you have to change pen colors more often that way.)

CHARTING WITH INSTRUMENTS WITH M.E.N.S. SERIES METERS

Dr. Greenlee has simplified meridian charting by designing a new grid with more space. Now, rather than using a line to designate readings, we write the numbers. Differences of ten points are considered splits (on the older charts, splits were indicated by differences of twenty points). To rechart, simply skip a line and record the new numbers on the next line.

For the sake of those practitioners still using instruments with older meters, most of the examples in the following section are illustrated with the line method of charting, however we have included some examples of the new charts along with a master sheet that may be duplicated as needed. We recommend also making copies of the Common Points Chart on page 155 for quick reference when balancing meridians.

This section on REL is only applicable to those using older instruments.

RELATIVE ENERGY LEVEL

REL are the initials Dr. Wing gave to represent the overall energy or "chi" of the patient. It is relative to the patient as an individual, not to the general populace. The percentage the patient is deficient or excessive relates to the amount of energy the patient usually has. In the Chinese concept, women are considered yin and men are yang. This is normal. A woman on the yang side might find her energy restless, nervous. She might be driven, but find little satisfaction, be constantly agitated, yet accomplish little. It's the wheel-spinning condition which leaves one exhausted. A man on the yang side would be all right. An excess of yang, however, might give him the same symptoms as the REL + woman. An REL - man would be devoid of energy. A woman can be at -35 and still feel all right.

CALCULATING REL

REL is calculated once all the meridian levels have been recorded. Dr. Wing obtains his REL by adding together all the meridian readings and then dividing by the number of the meridians measured. Dr. Greenlee lays a ballpoint pen or pencil across the chart where the majority of readings fall. To determine his treatments, he notes whatever shows above or below it. Where the tip of the pencil points is the REL reading. This, he says, is the advanced method of determining REL. By recording the REL before and after each therapy, you can see by the differences in readings the effectiveness of whatever changes you have made in therapy. This can be chiropractic adjustment, physical therapy, vitamins, diet, exercise, etc.. Dr. Wing recommends measuring the REL on the next visit prior to any therapy, and then comparing it to the previous REL to determine the effectiveness of therapy.

INTERPRETING CHARTS

In the next section, Dr. Greenlee takes you through a number of charts to help you understand what to look for and how to approach what you find. First you will see the former method of charting, then the new method. In the former, Dr. Greenlee's REL references are based on a scale where Zero is at the darkened horizontal center line in the middle of the chart. All readings above it are considered + (Plus); all below are considered to be - (Minus) in increments of ten points.

Correct procedures will tend to bring the meridian readings closer together. This is especially true with adjustive procedures. These readouts can provide a way to monitor the patient's progress, both immediately and over a long period of time.

SIGNIFICANCE OF MERIDIAN CHARTS

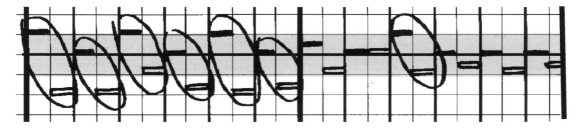

splits between right and left sides

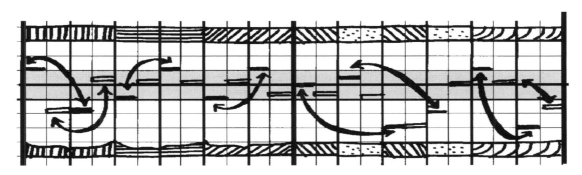

splits between Coupled Meridians (front and back of body)

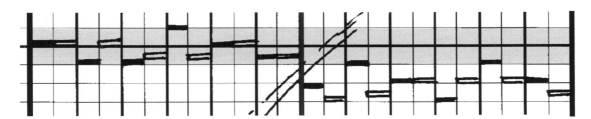

splits between upper and lower parts of the body

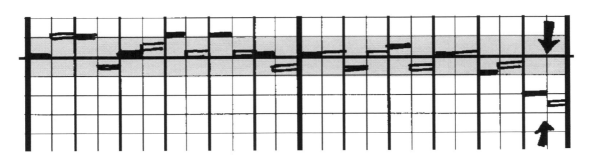

specific meridian problems

PROTOCOL OF INTERPRETATION

1. Relative Energy Level.

Low readings mean low energy flow, high readings, high energy flow. It gives indication of the body's ability to respond. For low energy, it may be necessary to check and correct the condition before the electrical treatments will be effective.

2. Normal

A normal chart will show all the readings between the right and left sides to be the same. On the charts, a ten point difference is acceptable.

3. Splits

Differences of more than ten points between the right and left on the same meridians are called splits. Minor splits usually correct when the major problems within the charts are corrected. Differences of more than twenty points between right and left are considered major splits.

Imbalances between left and right tell us if there is a dominance of one side over the other. This is particularly evident in stroke victims, and more subtle in cases of cross dominance where there is constant tension in the nervous system because the person is left-dominant and uses his right hand. There is a psychological significance relating to the functions of the yin and yang brains. Left dominance indicates more energy in the emotional side. It also indicates parasympathetic dominance.

The following are patient charts.

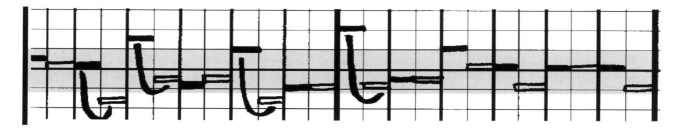

If one side is dominant, particularly in the upper meridians, it is usually indicative of the need for an atlas adjustment, though it could also be axis or condyles.

4. Switching

Switching is indicated through the presence of major splits on right and left where sometimes the right side is higher and sometimes the left. It demonstrates a neurological switching with the body. If there are more than five meridians involved, it normally indicates a problem of a cranial mandibular (TMJ) lesion or a cranial fixation to be corrected. Other causes of switching are the use of marijuana and secondhand smoke.

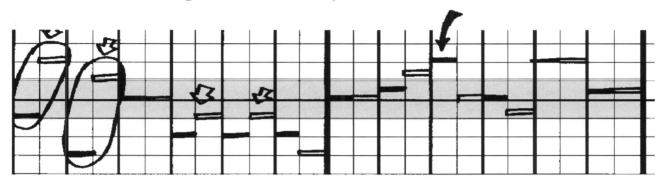

The following is a chart of the same patient as shown in the chart above. A TMJ adjustment changed the read out to this.

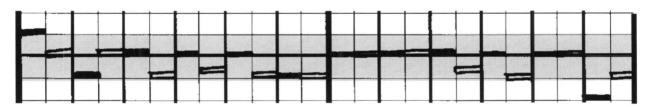

Unbalanced lower meridians often indicate dysfunction further down the spine.

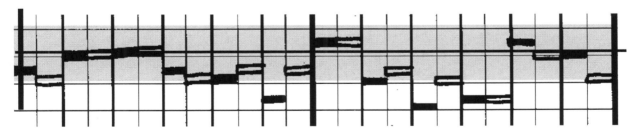

After a sacral adjustment, the patient looked like this.

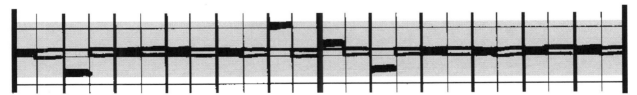

BALANCING WITH ADJUSTMENTS

There are many different ways to balance the meridians, but these three types of adjustments take precedence over the others. It is our experience that, unless these structural imbalances are corrected, meridians cannot hold their balance. Correct procedures will be reflected in the increasing balance of meridians on charts taken over a period of time.

More than five major and/or minor splits without change in dominance indicate the need for upper cervical correction.

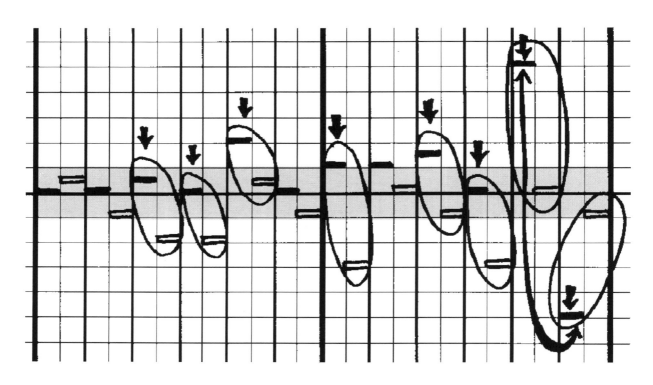

Atlas (before)

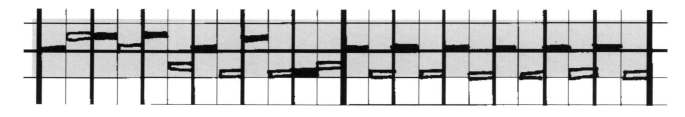

Atlas (after)

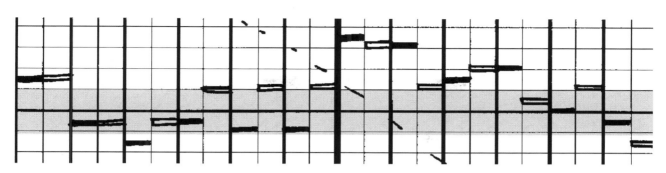

Sacrum (before)

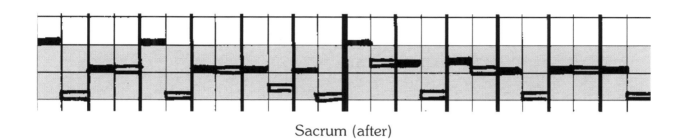

Sacrum (after)

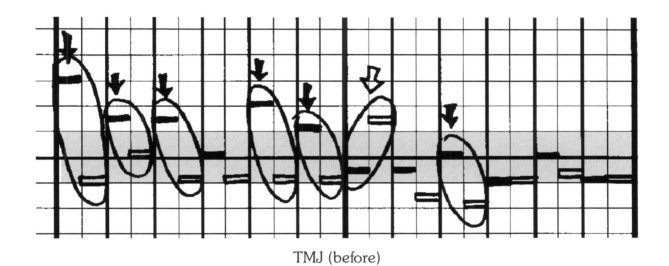

TMJ (before)

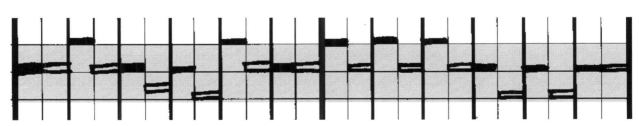

TMJ (after bilateral adjustment)

6. Splits mainly on the meridians which run through the hands

When the splits are primarily in the meridians which run through the hands, it is usually upper cervical involvement. However, if the majority of the splits are in the foot meridians, it will be subluxation or fixation between L4 and the sacrum.

7. Major splits on a single meridian or between Coupled Meridians (chiropractic interpretation)

Major splits on a single meridian or between Coupled Meridians (front and back) will be associated within the area of the vertebral points listed below for the specific meridians. Check the area of involvement for tenderness to determine the specific vertebrae. When considering the number of splits for adjusting purposes, splits in Coupled Meridians are counted as well as splits between right and left sides. There are no levels for the TH.

MERIDIAN	VERTEBRAL LEVEL
LU	T1, T2, T8, T9
LI	L2, L5
HC & HT	T2, T8, T12
SI	T12, L1, L5
SP	T1, T5, T9
LV	T2, T5, T8
ST	T8, T10, T12
GB	T4, T5
KI	T5, T8, L5, sacrum
BL	L5, sacrum

COUPLED MERIDIANS	
Metal:	LU & LI
Fire:	HC & TH
Fire:	HT & SI
Earth:	SP & ST
Wood:	LV & GB
Water:	KI & BL

8. Splits in single meridians

Splits in single meridians need also to be evaluated with splits within yin and yang meridians of each meridian element, such as the difference of twenty points between LU and LI, both in the element Metal. Also look for right and left splits between yin and yang elements.

BALANCING MERIDIANS WITH ACUPOINTS

After taking a meridian read out, circle the splits. If there are quite a few, you will probably have to do some sort of manipulation before you can do any more balancing. If no manipulation is possible, follow the procedures on p. 99 at the end of this section. After all basic splits are corrected, there may be one or two meridians still out of balance. At this point, you are fine tuning or treating a specific organ or system point which has not been corrected by spinal adjusting.

Evaluation of meridian imbalances within all the meridians requires more knowledge than this book supplies, however the following procedures, which I've worked out according to acupuncture laws, will give you, in most cases, the desired results--which is that the meridian measurements on the chart be within ten points of one another on new instruments (the M.E.N.S. II, IV or M.E.N.S.-i Super) or twenty on the old.

When searching for acupoints, remember that patients don't perfectly match the models. Even among standard acupuncture charts there may be discrepancies of one or two points. Go for the tender points. Also, keep in mind the golf principle: the current will flow to the lowest point. With needle acupuncture, you have to be specific, but not with microcurrent. Use these settings on the points recommended in this section:

Hertz:	10 Hz	**Wave Slope:**	Medium
Microamps:	40–100 μA	**Time:**	10–15 seconds

1. Following correction of splits, check for most yin meridian. Tonify both sides and recheck. Use the Five Element Tonification Points in the order listed on the chart on p. 90. They have been worked out by Dr. Felix Mann according to each stimulation's effect on other organs. Yang tends to follow yin. That means when you put the energy in the yin meridian, it tends to correct the yang meridian at the same time. This is a quick and efficient way to correct charts that are not greatly out of balance. When you are instructed to treat "the Tonification Point," use the first point listed for the meridian.

2. For a single excessive meridian, you may use Five Element Sedation Points in the order listed on page 90. When instructed to treat "the Sedation Point," use only the first point listed for the meridian.

   Charts showing the location of the points are on pages 92 and 93.

FIVE ELEMENT SEDATION POINTS

LUNG	LU 5	KI 10	LU 10	HT 8
LARGE INTESTINE	LI 2	BL 66	LI 5	SI 5
STOMACH	ST 45	LI 1	ST 43	GB 41
SPLEEN	SP 5	LU 8	SP 1	LV 1
HEART	HT 7	SP 3	HT 3	KI 10
SMALL INTESTINE	SI 8	ST 36	SI 2	BL 66
BLADDER	BL 65	GB 41	BL 54	ST 36
KIDNEY	KI 1	LV 1	KI 3	SP 3
HEART CONSTRICTOR	HC 7	SP 3	HC 3	KI 10
TRI HEATER	TH 10	ST 36	TH 2	BL 66
GALLBLADDER	GB 38	SI 5	GB 44	LI 1
LIVER	LV 2	HT 8	LV 4	LU 8

FIVE ELEMENT TONIFICATION POINTS

LUNG	LU 9	SP 3	LU 10	HT 8
LARGE INTESTINE	LI 11	ST 36	LI 5	SI 5
HEART CONSTRICTOR	HC 9	LV 1	HC 3	KI 10
TRI HEATER	TH 3	GB 41	TH 2	BL 66
HEART	HT 9	LV 1	HT 3	KI 10
SMALL INTESTINE	SI 3	GB 41	SI 2	BL 66
SPLEEN	SP 2	HT 8	SP 1	LV 1
LIVER	LV 8	KI 10	LV 4	LU 8
STOMACH	ST 41	SI 5	ST 43	GB 41
GALLBLADDER	GB 43	BL 66	GB 44	LI 1
KIDNEY	KI 7	LU 8	KI 3	SP 3
BLADDER	BL 67	LI 1	BL 54	ST 36

3. Imbalances between meridians within the element:

Use meridian LUO POINT on the side of the excess to send the energy from the high side to the low.

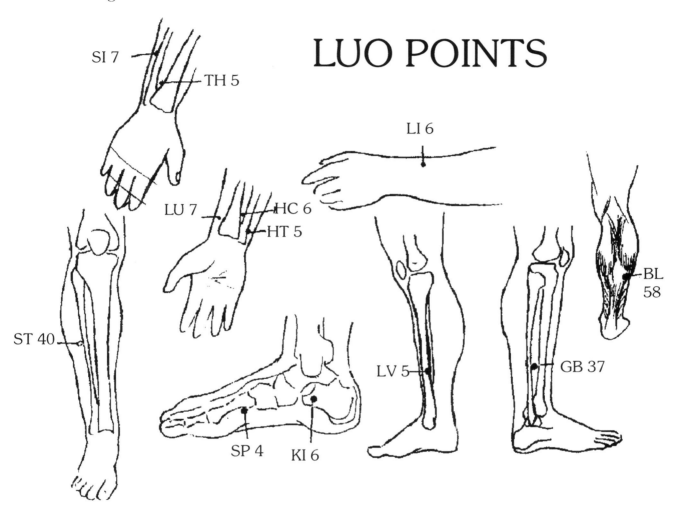

LUO POINTS

Luo Points are the bridges between Coupled Meridians, such as Stomach/Spleen, Kidney/Bladder. They are also known as "Coupling Points" or "Connecting Points" because that's what they do. To transfer energy, always use the Luo Point on the excessive meridian.

Luo Points are as follows:
    LU 7, LI 6, LV 5, ST 40, SP 4, GB 37, HT 5, BL 58, TH 5, KI 4, HC 6.

We used to recommend using the Luo Point on the side of deficiency to draw energy to the low meridian, but we have found it more powerful to send energy from the excessive to the deficient.

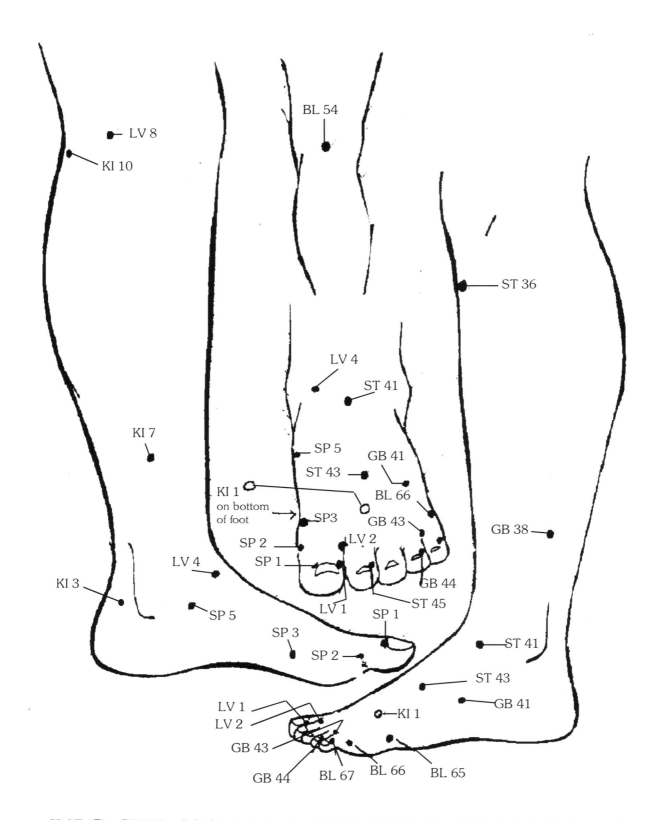

BL 54

LV 8

KI 10

ST 36

KI 7

LV 4

ST 41

SP 5

GB 41

ST 43

KI 1
on bottom
of foot

BL 66

SP3

GB 43

SP 2

LV 2

GB 38

LV 4

SP 1

KI 3

GB 44

SP 5

ST 45

LV 1

SP 1

SP 3

ST 41

SP 2

ST 43

LV 1

GB 41

LV 2

KI 1

GB 43

GB 44

BL 67

BL 66

BL 65

LEG SEDATION & TONIFICATION POINTS

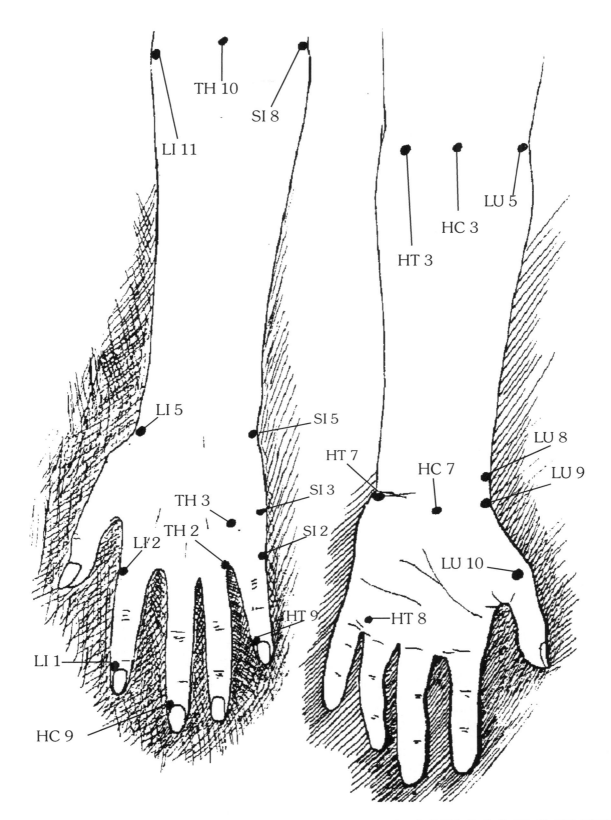

ARM TONIFICATION & SEDATION POINTS

93

4. You may also clean up small deficiencies with SOURCE POINTS.

    All Source Points are localized in the wrist or ankle. They serve when a disequilibrium of energy in a meridian is accompanied by organic symptoms. They may also be used when associated with organ dysfunction as noted by scanning auricular points.

    These points have a direct effect on the organs that correspond to the meridians from which they take their names. Example: The lung Source Point would directly affect the lung.

    If the meridian is yin, the Source Point will be the meridian's EARTH point:

    LU 9, SP 3, HT 7, KI 3, HC 7, LV 3...

    Source Points for the yang meridians are distinctive and not associated with the elements. They seem to have a specific intimacy with the organs:

    LI 4, ST 42, SI 4, BL 64, TH 4, GB 40.

5. When general energy is excessive (the majority of points above 75 on the new meter), the patient will feel agitated or totally fatigued. The procedure for balancing this kind of excessive energy is in the section on Hand Acupoint Therapy on p. 133.

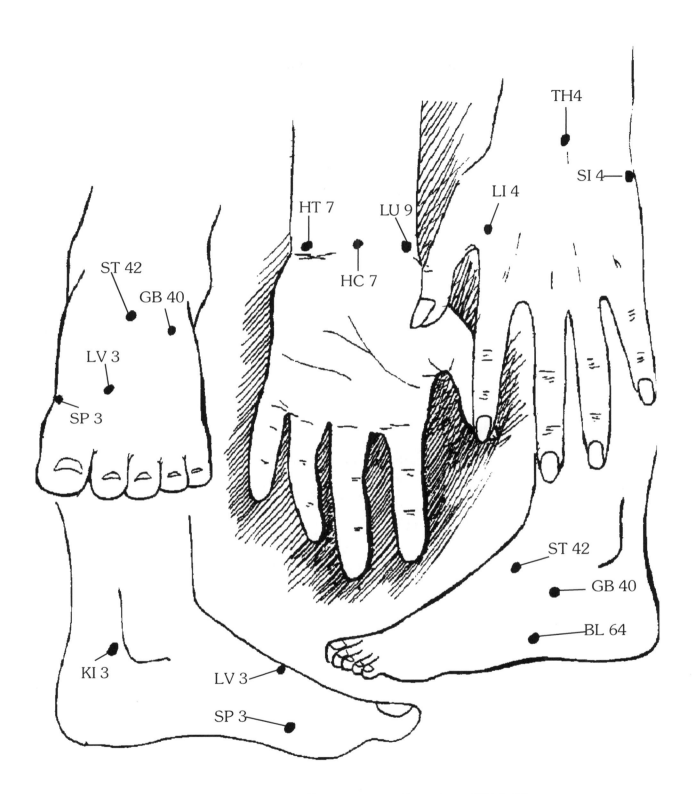

SOURCE POINTS

95

6. If energy is fairly even but low, use MASTER POINTS. They are safe to use most any time except in cases of extreme yang REL. They raise energy and balance at the same time. When in doubt, use Master Points (except yang REL).

MASTER POINTS

SP6--3 cun* above the top of the medial malleolus just posterior to tibial border. Measure 4 fingers up from ankle bone
*cur human inch—roughly the distance between first and second joints of the index finger

BL 54--exact midpoint of popliteal transverse crease

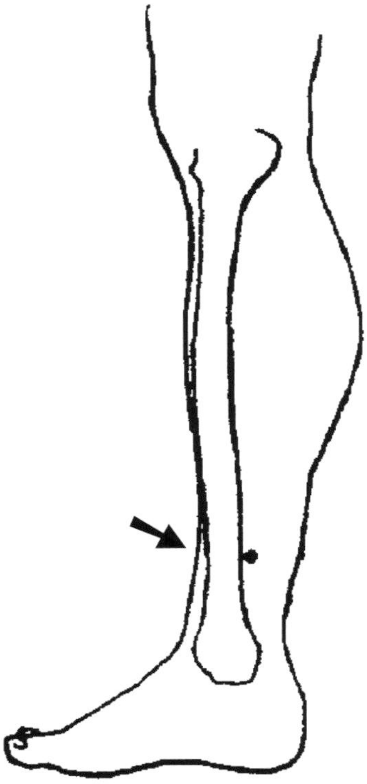

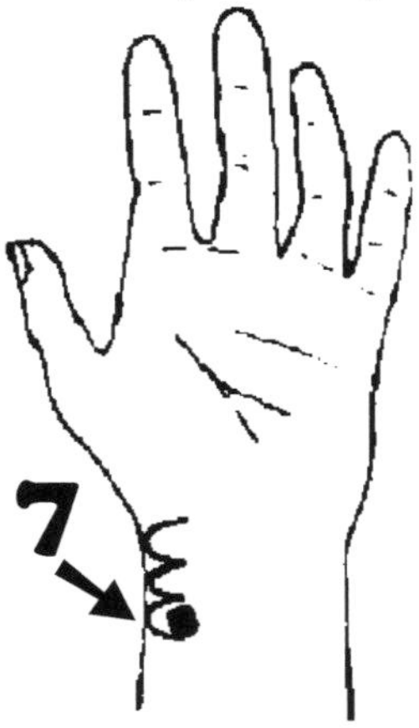

LU 7

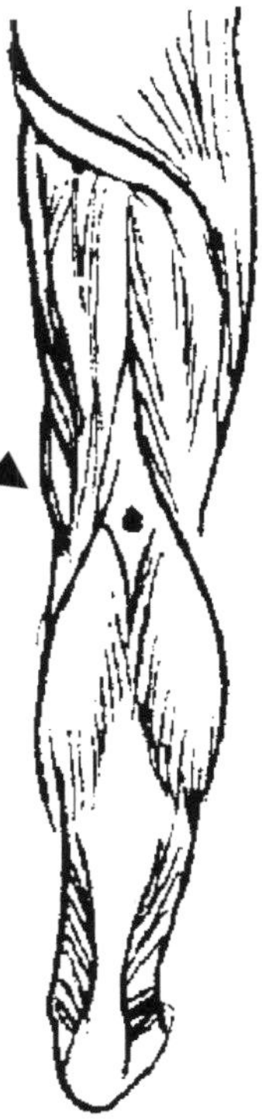

SP 6

LI 4

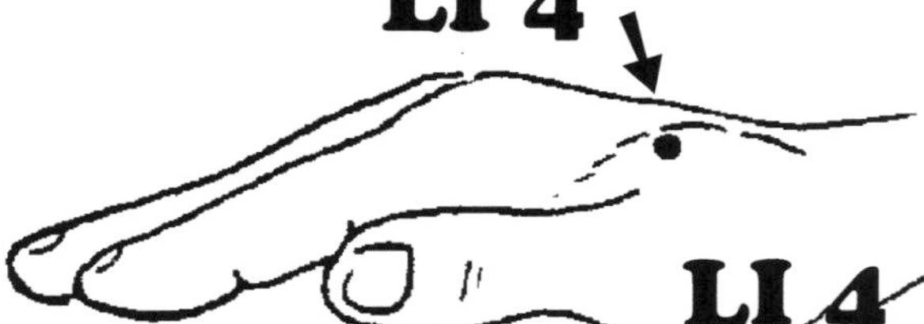

BL 54

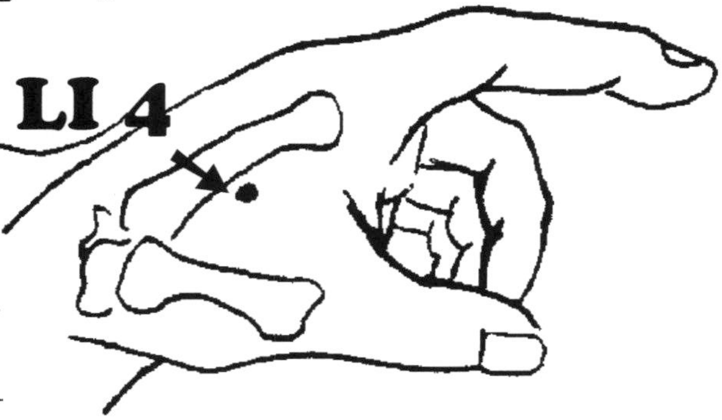

LU 7--3 fingers up from wrist

LI 4--on the middle of the second metacarpal bone, on the radial aspect. Also at the highest spot on the muscle when thumb and index finger are brought close together.

LI 4

ST 36--1 finger breadth from the anterior crest of the tibia

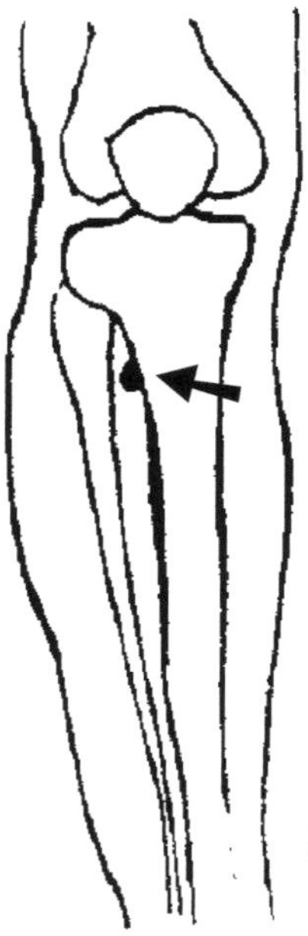

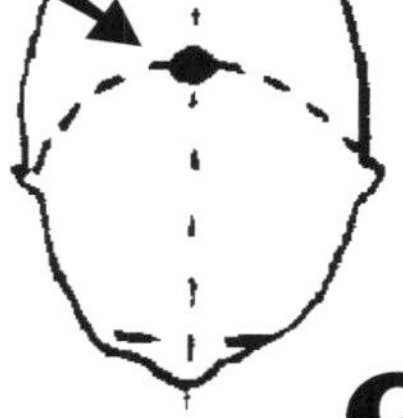

GV 20--intersection of ears and nose on top of head

ST 36

Alternate Master Points:
SP 6, ST 36, LI 4, LU 7

GV 20

7. Small deficiencies can also be handled with EAR POINTS. We believe ear points help normalize the problem.

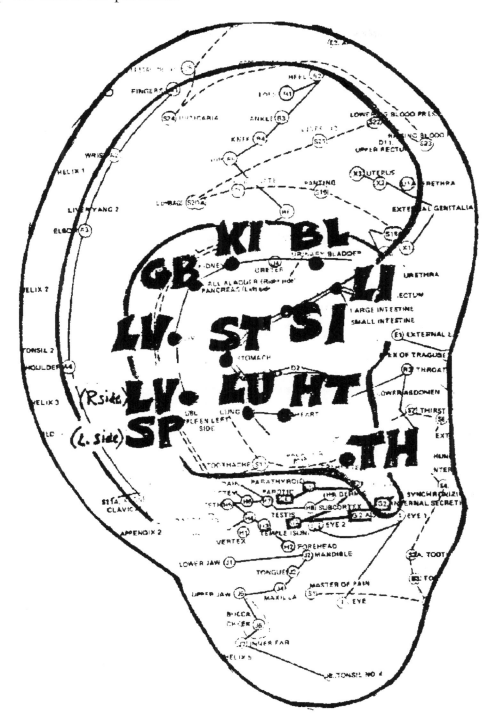

EAR POINTS CORRESPONDING TO MERIDIANS

8. For small imbalances, use ASSOCIATE POINTS. They can also be used as a general tonic. Associate Points are located within the Bladder meridian located along the spine. They are related to each of the twelve meridians and associated with the organs from which the meridians draw their names. In classic acupuncture, they are considered Reflex Points.

Associate Points may be used diagnostically. If they are tender upon light palpation, the meridian or organ is underactive. If they are tender to deep palpation, the meridian or organ is overactive.

Lower resistance to electrical stimulation is significant in helping to locate imbalances (shown by higher readings on the meter and higher pitch). Treatment of these points is also effective in dealing with associated organ problems.

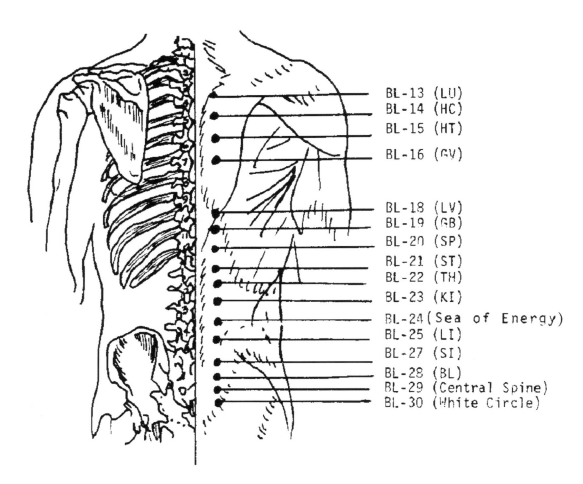

BL-13 (LU)
BL-14 (HC)
BL-15 (HT)
BL-16 (GV)

BL-18 (LV)
BL-19 (GB)
BL-20 (SP)
BL-21 (ST)
BL-22 (TH)
BL-23 (KI)
BL-24 (Sea of Energy)
BL-25 (LI)
BL-27 (SI)
BL-28 (BL)
BL-29 (Central Spine)
BL-30 (White Circle)

ASSOCIATE POINTS

IF NO ADJUSTMENT IS POSSIBLE

If no adjustment is possible, first use T.E.S.T. through the vertebral area which would normally be adjusted using double Qs, 3-D probes or MQ-6s.

For upper cervical splits, T.E.S.T. bilaterally through the upper cervical spine under the skull. Stimulate GV 20 and KI 27 bilaterally (KI 27 is found at the sternal costal clavicular junction).

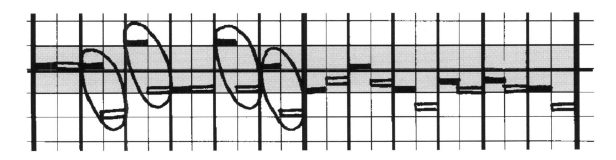

In lower extremities, T.E.S.T. through lumbosacral area.

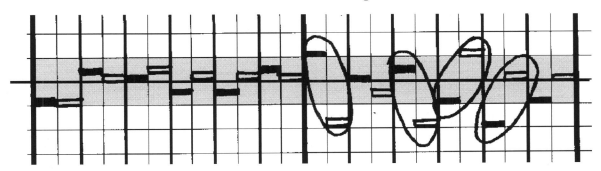

Splits between upper and lower extremities, T.E.S.T. through Associate Points in lower dorsal and upper lumbar regions.

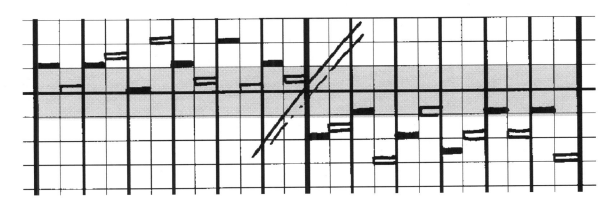

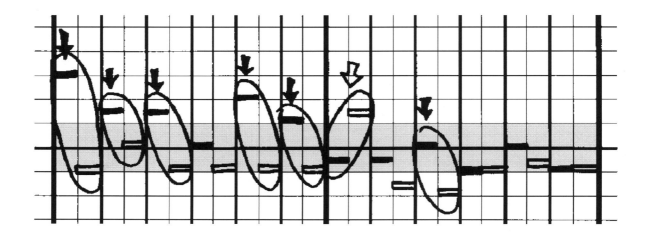

For switching (splits with change of dominance),
T.E.S.T. through the TMJ areas and follow with Master Points.

For individual splits, T.E.S.T. through the vertebral level indicated
by the splits and follow with Master Points.

MERIDIAN	VERTEBRAL LEVEL
LUNG	T1, T2, T8, T9
LARGE INTESTINE	L2, L5
HEART CONSTRICTOR & HEART	T2, T8, T12
SMALL INTESTINE	T12, L1, L5
SPLEEN	T1, T5, T9
LIVER	T2, T5, T8
STOMACH	T8, T10, T12
GALLBLADDER	T4, T5
KIDNEY	T5, T8, L5, sacrum
BLADDER	L5, sacrum

EXAMPLES & TREATMENT OPTIONS

In these examples, Dr. Greenlee indicates what he looks for when evaluating a meridian chart and offers suggestions on treatment.

CHART A

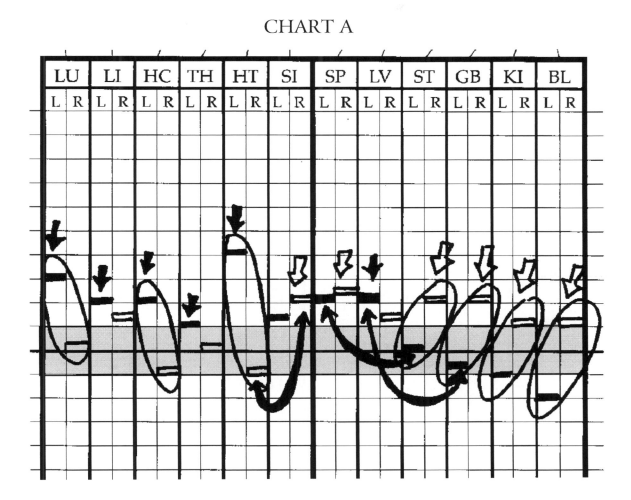

1. Splits Between Right and Left Sides

   A. Multiple splits between left and right on the following meridians:
      LU, HC, HT, ST, GB, KI, BL
   B. Splits between left sides of the following Coupled Meridians:
      HT & SI
      SP & ST
      LV & GB
   C. Splits between right side of HT and SI

   These splits indicate the need for an upper cervical adjustment.

Change of Dominance (Switching)
  A. Left dominance on the following meridians:
      LU, LI, HC, HT, LV
  B. Right dominance on the following meridians:
      SI, SP, ST, GB, KI, BL

TREATMENT OPTIONS
  • Upper cervical adjustment and/or cranial adjustment
  • TMJ correction
  • If manipulative procedures are not possible, T.E.S.T. through upper cervical verte-
    bra and along the skull bilaterally
  • For switching, stimulate GV 20 and KI 27 bilaterally with 20 Hz, 100 μA, 10
  seconds.
  • Use Tonification Point on right side of HT.

CHART B

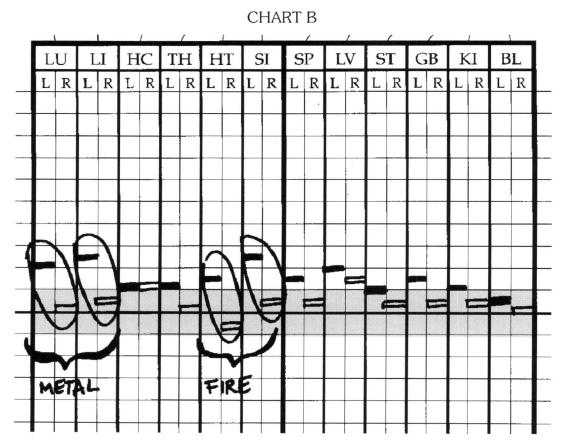

1. Major splits on hand meridians.
2. Splits between right and left sides of meridians within the same element.

TREATMENT OPTIONS:
  • Correct with upper cervical adjustment.
  • T.E.S.T. through upper cervical vertebrae and along the base of the skull.

102

CHART C

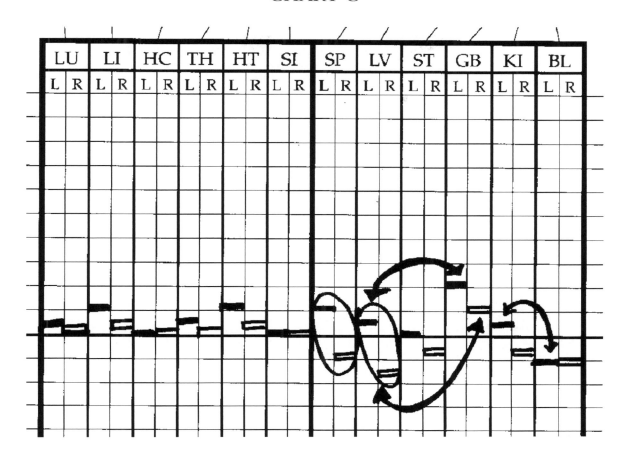

LU		LI		HC		TH		HT		SI		SP		LV		ST		GB		KI		BL	
L	R	L	R	L	R	L	R	L	R	L	R	L	R	L	R	L	R	L	R	L	R	L	R

1. Major splits on foot meridians
2. Major splits between right and left sides within the following meridians:
   SP, LV
3. Right and left split (right side) within the elements of the following meridians:
   LV, GB
4. Right and left split (left side) within the elements of the following meridians:
   KI, BL

TREATMENT OPTIONS:
- Adjust L4, L5 and sacrum
- T.E.S.T. through vertebral area

CHART D

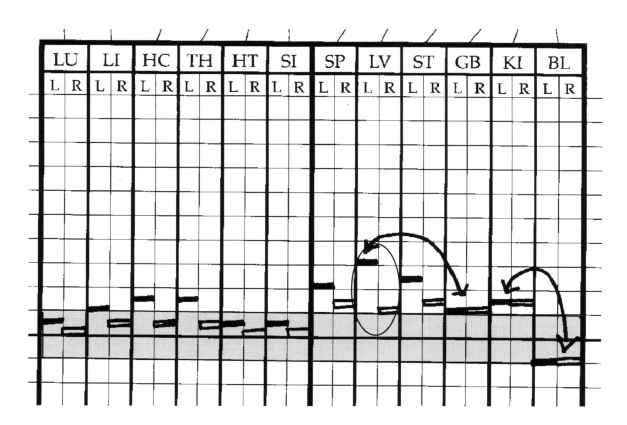

1. Splits on an individual meridian—LV
2. Splits within coupled meridians on the following meridians:
   LV, GB and KI, BL

TREATMENT OPTIONS

- Treat corresponding thoracic for GB and LV: T2, T5, T8
- Treat LV with right LV Luo point
- For KI and BL there are several possibilities:
—Bilateral BL Luo points (always use Luo Points on the deficient side)
—Bilateral Tonification Points on BL to elevate BL (The reason for not sedating
    KI is because that would have no effect on the BL)
—Use BL Five Element Points for tonification

CHART E

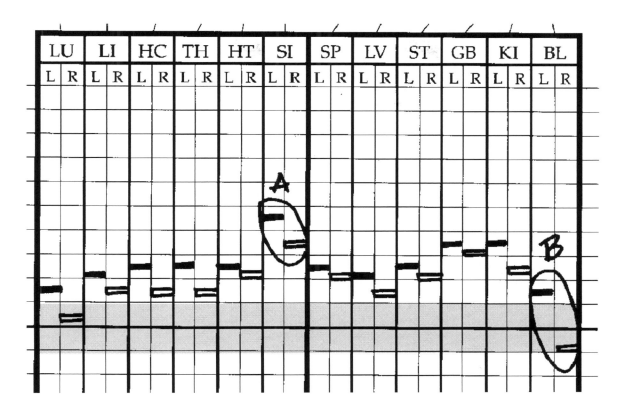

LU		LI		HC		TH		HT		SI		SP		LV		ST		GB		KI		BL	
L	R	L	R	L	R	L	R	L	R	L	R	L	R	L	R	L	R	L	R	L	R	L	R

A. Note the following:
1. The higher readings on the SI meridian
2. A split on the left sides of Coupled Meridians HT and SI
3. The left side of SI is elevated above most other meridians

TREATMENT OPTIONS
- Adjustment of corresponding vertebral area for SI
- Bilateral Luo points on HT (not likely to work by itself)
- Bilateral single Sedation Point on SI
- Bilateral Five Element Sedation Points on the SI
  I would use first the Luo Point on the low side of SI, then the Five Element Sedation Points to regulate energy of the other meridians to compensate for the movement of energy.
- Auricular points for SI

B. Note the following:
1. Right BL point is lower than all the others
2. Meridian splits between left KI and BL
3. Meridian splits between right KI and BL
4. Minor split between right and left sides of BL

TREATMENT OPTIONS
- Adjustment of L5 and sacrum
- Tonification Point of right BL.
- I would not use the Luo Point because I don't want the energy to come down to the right BL
- Five Element Tonification Points on the BL right side; this is the preferable choice

CHART F

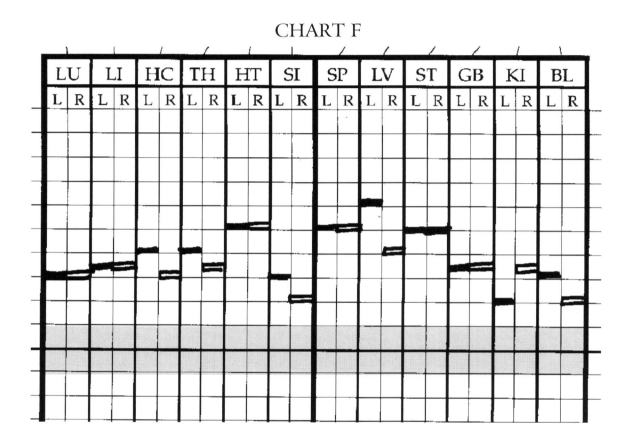

1. On hand points, there is a bilateral split on the Coupled Meridian of HT and SI.
2. On the foot points, there is a right and left meridian split on the LV.
3. Between the Coupled Meridians of LV and GB, there is a left side split.
4. There is a minor split between the right KI and BL Coupled Meridians.
5. The Coupled Meridian of SP and ST are level, but they are also higher than the rest.

TREATMENT OPTIONS
- Thoracic adjustment T2, T4, T5.
- For LV split, use LV Luo Point.
- For KI, BL split, use right BL Luo Point.
- The treatment of the high SP and ST will need to be reconsidered, or auricular points may be used.

CHART G

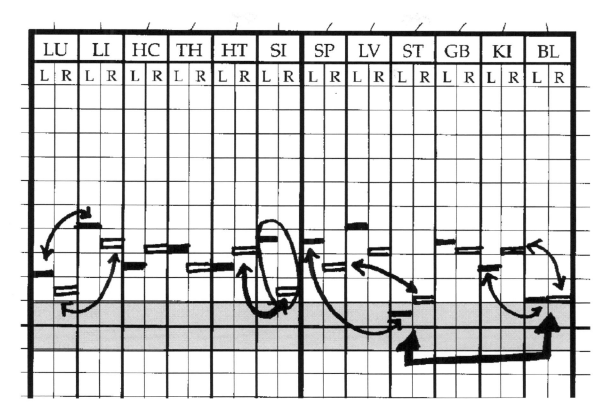

LU		LI		HC		TH		HT		SI		SP		LV		ST		GB		KI		BL	
L	R	L	R	L	R	L	R	L	R	L	R	L	R	L	R	L	R	L	R	L	R	L	R

1. Splits on left and right of SI
2. Coupled splits left and right LU and LI, KI and BL, SP and ST, right HT and SI
3. Marked difference in ST and BL
4. Changes of dominance in HC, HT, ST and KI

TREATMENT OPTIONS

For multiple splits (5 meridians and on coupled)
- Upper cervical treatment
- TMJ treatment

Should rechart after adjustment and then consider other options.

For LU and LI split
- Bilateral Luo Points
- Bilateral Tonification Points
- Five Element Tonification Points

For splits between right HT and right SI
- Right SI Luo Point
- Right Tonification or Source Point on SI

For split between SP and ST meridians

Since treatment objective is to raise energy to correspond with energy of the other meridians, use bilateral Source Points, Tonification Points, or Five Element Tonification Points. The treatment of choice is the Five Element Tonification Points.

For split between KI and BL
- Bilateral Tonification Points
- Bilateral Source Points
- Five Element Points

Note: as a rule, if you choose to use Five Element Tonification Points on the most deficient meridian, it is not usually necessary to treat each specific problem since the Five Element Points tend to correct all the meridians.

THINGS TO CONSIDER WITH MERIDIAN BALANCE

Akabane balancing is primarily looking at the musculo-tendon system of the body and its possible responses to the corresponding viscera. It is primarily responding to the area that the viscera influence, so this becomes an objective finding and needs to always be considered and confirmed with other findings.

When dealing with energy, it is always best to move energy from where there is excess to the deficient, therefore, when choosing balancing procedures, try to move the energy and not sedate it. Localized sedation of pain is not like sedating in the movement of system energy.

FOR BALANCING WITH HAND ACUPOINTS, SEE PAGES. 133, 134

EVALUATING CHARTS

Order of Evaluation:

1. Look for splits between right and left sides within an individual meridian.
    These usually denote vertebral subluxations.

2. Look for right and left splits between coupled meridians.
    These usually denote vertebral subluxations.

3. Look for splits between coupled meridians (yin and yang meridians within each element). These usually denote vertebral subluxations.

4. Check for change of dominance within splits (switching).
    More than three usually means there are TMJ or cranial fixations.

4. Check for meridians with highest and lowest readings.

5. Make note of the yin merdians with the lowest readings.

Suggested Methods of Correction:

Splits between the right and left sides of individual meridians may be corrected by using the Luo Point on the high side or by using the the Tonification or Source Points on the low sides of the meridians.

Splits between coupled meridians may be corrected by using the Luo Point on the right and left sides of the high meridian or the Tonification or Source Points on the right and left sides of the low meridians.

Single meridian deficiency may be corrected with Tonification Points or Source Points.

Single excessive meridians may be corrected with Sedation Points (seldom used).

Multiple imbalances within the meridians may be treated with Five Element Points.
~Use the Five Element Points for sedation and tonification as found on page 90 or
~Draw the energy from the most excessive meridian to the most deficient.

Use the Element Point on the most excessive meridian to "turn the meridian on."
Then choose the same element point on the deficient meridian and stimulate.

Element Points are listed on the Common Points chart on page 155.

Examples:

SP is excessive. SP's element is Earth. Use the SP Earth Point (SP3) first.

BL is deficient. Draw energy from Earth by using the BL Earth Point BL 54.

If there are no specific excesses, treat the most yin meridian with the first Tonification Point on the chart on p. 90. But if there are many symptoms, use all four Tonification Points in the order listed.

The following are examples of how to read charts using Dr. Greenlee's notation system.

CHART W

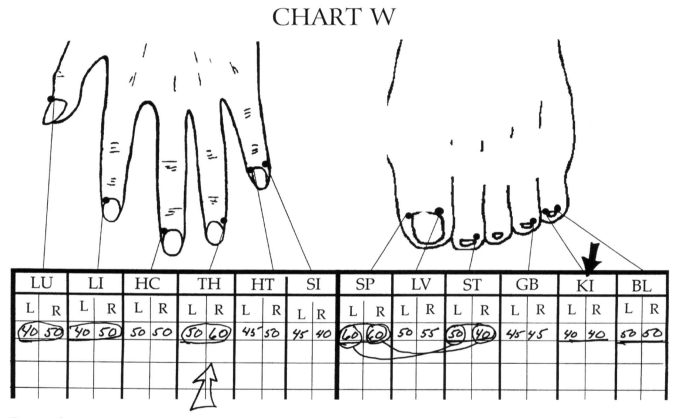

LU		LI		HC		TH		HT		SI		SP		LV		ST		GB		KI		BL	
L	R	L	R	L	R	L	R	L	R	L	R	L	R	L	R	L	R	L	R	L	R	L	R
40	50	40	50	50	50	50	60	45	50	45	40	60	60	50	55	50	40	45	45	40	40	50	50

Procedure:

Check each meridian for splits between left and right sides and circle: LU, LI, TH, ST.

Circle and connect splits on coupled meridians, left to left, right to right: left SP to left ST, right SP to right ST.

Underline splits between coupled meridians: KI and BL.

Find the most excessive meridian: SP.

Find the most deficient yin organ: KI.

CHART X

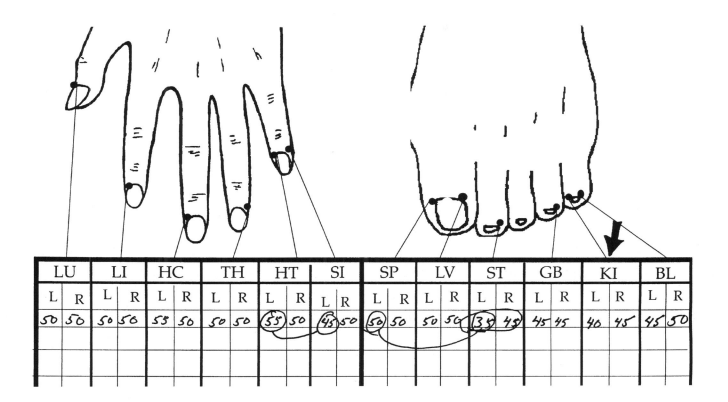

LU		LI		HC		TH		HT		SI		SP		LV		ST		GB		KI		BL	
L	R	L	R	L	R	L	R	L	R	L	R	L	R	L	R	L	R	L	R	L	R	L	R
50	50	50	50	53	50	50	50	55	50	45	50	50	50	50	50	35	45	45	45	40	45	45	50

Procedure:

Circle splits between left and right sides within meridians: ST

Circle and connect splits between left and right sides of coupled meridians: left of HT and SI, left of SP and ST.

Note excessive meridians: none on this chart

Note most deficient yin meridian: KI

CHART Y

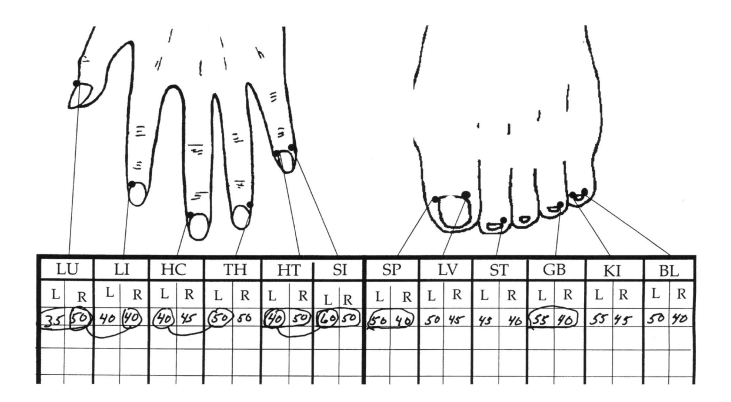

LU		LI		HC		TH		HT		SI		SP		LV		ST		GB		KI		BL	
L	R	L	R	L	R	L	R	L	R	L	R	L	R	L	R	L	R	L	R	L	R	L	R
35	50	40	40	40	45	50	50	40	50	60	50	50	40	50	45	43	46	55	40	55	45	50	40

Procedure:

Circle right and left splits within individual meridians: LU, HT, SI, SP, GB.

Circle and connect right and left splits between coupled meridians: left of HC and TH, left of HT and SI, right of LU and LI.

Note changes in dominance in coupled meridians: right side LU-LI, left side HC-TH, left side HT-SI. This may indicate atlas or spinal subluxation, TMJ or cranial lesions.

CHART Z

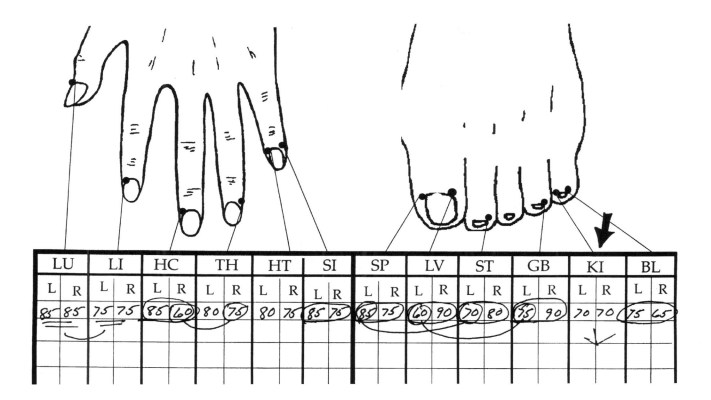

LU		LI		HC		TH		HT		SI		SP		LV		ST		GB		KI		BL	
L	R	L	R	L	R	L	R	L	R	L	R	L	R	L	R	L	R	L	R	L	R	L	R
85	85	75	75	85	60	80	75	80	75	85	75	85	75	60	90	70	80	75	90	70	70	75	65

Procedure:

Circle right and left splits within individual meridians: HC, SI, SP, LV, ST, GB, BL

Circle and connect right and left splits between coupled meridians: right to right: HC-TH, left to left: SP-ST, LV-GB

Underline splits between coupled meridians: LU-LI

Note the excessive readings on most of the meridians. This indicates yang excess. The individual may be excessively hyper or have total fatigue.

Find most deficient yin meridian: KI

EVALUATING THERAPY

If the procedures you are using are right for your patient, the splits and imbalances in his meridian charts will tend to move towards the normal range. This can happen over a period of time, or right away. With adjustive procedures, you will probably see immediate improvement, but sometimes acupuncture and other procedures take more time. Health does not return in a steady progression of happy ameliorations. Sometimes retracing makes the patient feel worse for awhile.

Don't be intimidated. While a wrong adjustment can definitely make a patient worse, treating with microcurrent is not so unforgiving. Even if you've read the charts wrong, any treatment given will tend to stir the pot and, in most instances, the body will seek homeostasis and the patient will get better. Don't be alarmed if, upon recharting, you see meridians in wild disarray (unless you've just given an adjustment). The meridians will generally settle down in an hour or so, and the next time the patient comes in, the new first chart will probably show more balance.

Anything that frees energy will tend to balance meridians. Conversely, anything that blocks it—traumas and insults to the system such as whiplash, white sugar, and rage—will throw them out of balance. You can tell your patients that, too. Hypoglycemics who cheat on their diets might show high Spleen energy and imbalance in the Liver and Gallbladder meridians. A person who has been coming to your office with fairly even charts should exhibit increased ability to hold that balance. If he comes in with splits when he has been coming balanced, he has blown his diet, messed up his bones, or had an emotional upset.

If you explain these charts to your patients, they will not only get the benefit of the immediate feedback, they might also begin taking responsibility for their own health.

The following series of charts shows S.W.'s progress through a number of procedures. These are all from the same day to show you what kind of balance is possible.

This is S.W.'s initial chart on her first visit to our office. The shaded area represents the center line. Her REL (if we had calculated it) would be -30. Notice the splits on the LI and GB meridians.

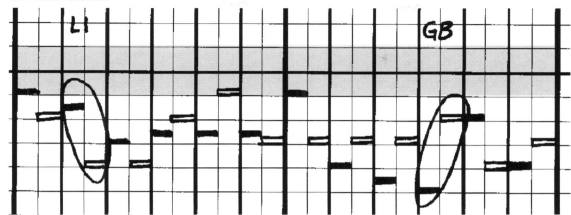

After a general adjustment, S.W.'s meridians lost their splits, came closer together, and her entire energy rose. The only meridians still out of balance are GB, KI and BL.

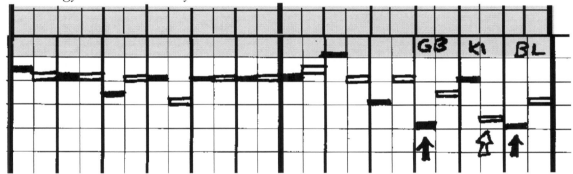

After stimulating BL Five Element Tonification Points at 20 Hz. for 8 seconds at 200 μA, S.W.'s energy level rose again and looked like this.

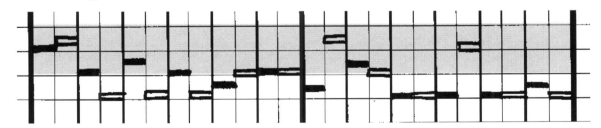

After stimulating Master Points bilaterally at 20 Hz. for 8 seconds at 200 μA, S.W.'s meridians came nearly into perfect balance.

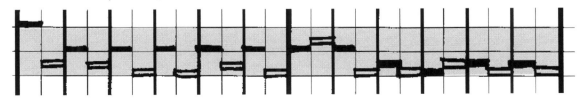

The following two charts show the change in the energy of this 43 year old woman from April to September. When S.W. first came in, she reported that she felt like wood from the waist down. Most of her reflexes were gone. She had to be practically carried in. She was diagnosed as having Lateral Sclerosis.

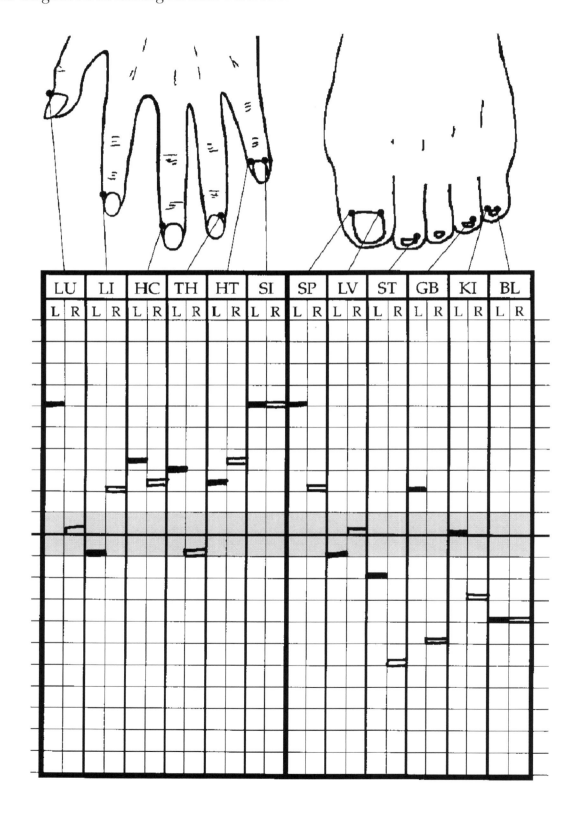

This woman went on a program of Logan Basic adjustments, meridian balancing, distilled water, nutritional supplementation, and a special diet. After five months, her charts looked like this, and continued in the same pattern each time she was rechecked at monthly intervals.

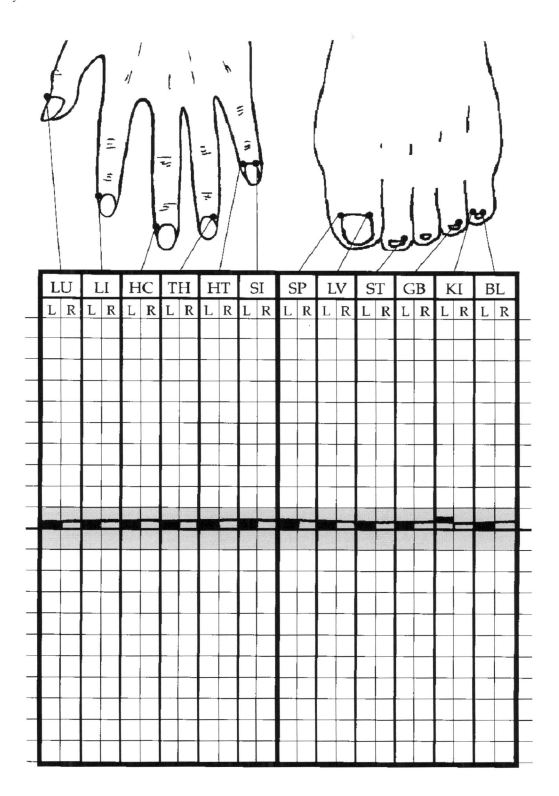

Greenlee Hand Chart

Name_____ Date_____ Time_____ a.m./p.m.

ST 4		SP 5		LV 5		HT 11		HC 10		LU 9		KI 3		BL 67		GB 30		LI 3		SI 3		TW 3	
L	R	L	R	L	R	L	R	L	R	L	R	L	R	L	R	L	R	L	R	L	R	L	R

KOREAN HAND ACUPOINT THERAPY

KOREAN HAND ACUPOINT THERAPY
by Dennis L. Greenlee, D.C., L.Ac.

Korean Hand Acupuncture was developed by Dr. Tae-Woo Yoo, OMD, Ph.D. Hand acupuncture is a complete system and can stand by itself. It is a holographic reiteration of the entire body which means that on each hand there is a correspondence to every area of the body including the entire meridian system. Nevertheless, the meridian system on the hands is not the same as the traditional body meridian points which are found on the hands. Each system stands by itself, but they can be used together to enhance the overall response picture.

Not only is there an anatomical correspondence found on each hand, there is also a functional correspondence. The meridian points on the hand also follow the basic laws of acupuncture and can be used in the same manner and with the same rules as acupuncture body points.

This text is an abbreviated application of the system as it relates to microcurrent. We will consider how to use microcurrent with Korean hand points to balance meridians, relieve pain, and treat specific organs. We'll be discussing tonification and sedation of meridians, corresponding points for treating specific organs and pain control.

Many times, even in this abbreviated approach, this therapy can stand alone. But the system as outlined in this book is usually used to support other procedures such as spinal correction, meridian balancing, and other systems of pain control. Note: Due to the power of this system, I highly recommend learning the entire system by attending Dr. Tae-Woo Yoo's seminars.

For the application of hand acupuncture points for meridian balancing, see p. 135.

Above: Large Intestine Body Meridian ~ Right: Large Intestine Hand Meridian

LARGE INTESTINE HAND MERIDIAN

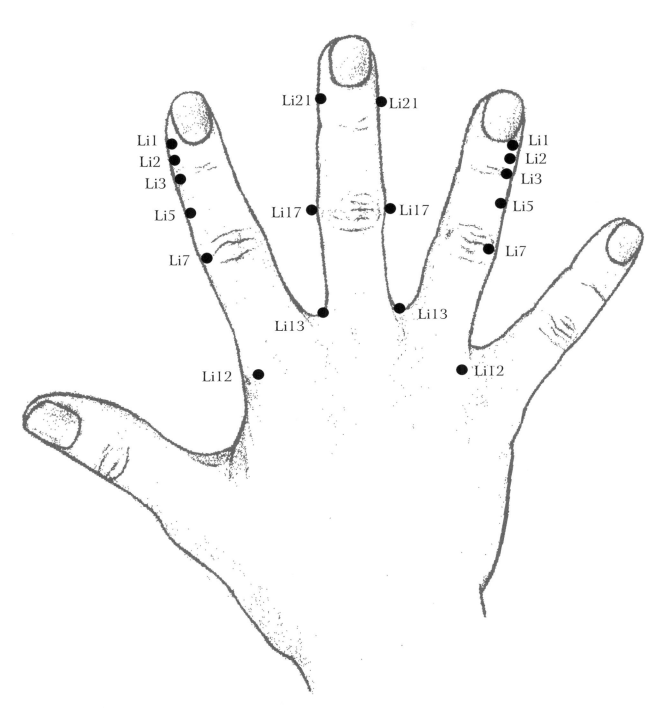

Notice that LI 4, a Master Point in Traditional Chinese Medicine, is not one of the points on the Large Intestine meridian of the Korean system.

MAKE UP OF THE HAND

Each hand singularly reflects the whole body. Upon the right hand, you can find corresponding points for any part of the whole body. Upon the left hand you can also find corresponding points for any part of the whole body. In other words you can treat the whole body on a single hand of a person. However, it is still best to treat the hand which is on the side of the dysfunction.

When looking at the back of a hand, note the middle finger as the division of the body between the right and the left sides, with the little finger representing the corresponding side of the body. In other words, on the right hand, the area from the right side of the middle finger to the little finger would represent the right side of the body. The left side of the middle finger to the thumb on the right hand would represent the left side of the body. Conversely, on the left hand, the left side of the middle finger to the little finger represents the left side of the body, and the right side of the middle finger to the thumb represents the right side of the body.

FINGER REPRESENTATION~BACK OF HAND

Middle finger on treating side=the spine
Tip of the finger to 1st knuckle=the head; first knuckle=occipital bone
First knuckle to the 2nd knuckle=neck; second knuckle=7th vertebra
Second knuckle to 3rd knuckle=upper thoracic vertebrae; third knuckle=7th thoracic vertebra

Third knuckle to the middle of the back of the hand=lower thoracic vertebrae
From the middle of the back of the hand to the flexion of the wrist =lumbar vertebrae
Joint of the wrist=lumbo-sacral joint

The ring finger=posterior side of upper extremity
From the tip of the finger to the first knuckle=hand, first knuckle being the wrist
From the first knuckle to the second knuckle=arm, with second knuckle being elbow
From the second knuckle to the third=upper arm, with third knuckle being shoulder

The little finger=posterior side of the lower extremity
From the tip of the finger to the first knuckle=foot, first knuckle being the ankle
From the first knuckle to second=lower leg, second knuckle being the knee
From the second knuckle to the third=thigh, third knuckle being the hip

The first finger=the posterior side of upper extremity on opposite side
Tip of the finger to first knuckle=hand, first knuckle being the wrist
From the first knuckle to the second knuckle=arm, with second knuckle being elbow
From the second knuckle to the third=upper arm, with third knuckle being shoulder

The thumb=posterior side of the lower extremity of the opposite side of the body.
Tip of thumb to first joint=foot, with first joint being ankle
From the first knuckle to the second= lower leg, second knuckle being the knee
From the second knuckle to base of thumb (junction of wrist and thumb)=thigh with
the base of the thumb being the hip

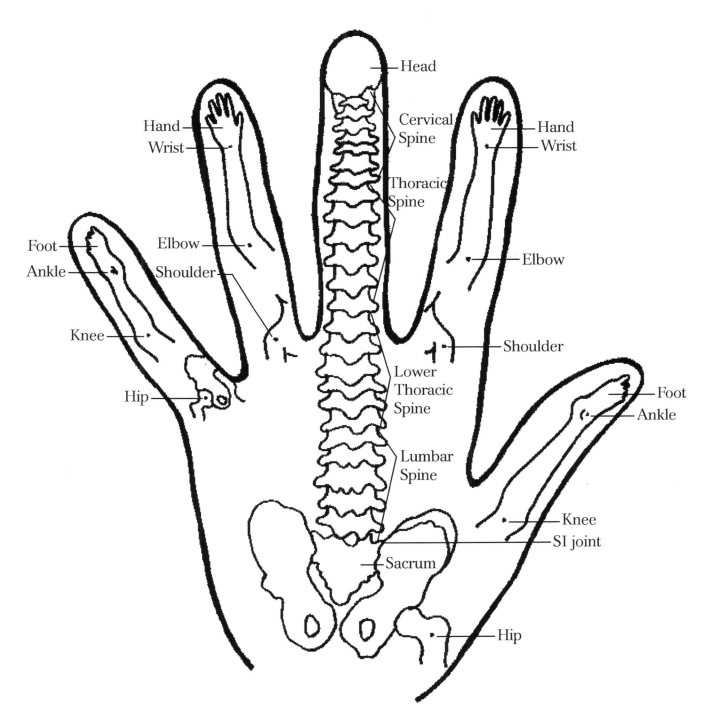

BACK OF HAND

FINGER REPRESENTATION~PALM OF HAND

On the palm of the hand, the middle finger represents the front of the torso, which includes the head, face, throat and chest. The palm of the hand is the abdominal cavity. The ring finger represents the palmer (yin) side of the hand, the wrist, elbow and shoulder. The little finger represents the anterior side of the foot, ankle, knee and hip. The 1st finger represents the hand, wrist, elbow and shoulder. The thumb represents the anterior side of the foot, ankle, knee, and hip on the opposite side of the body. As I stated before, it is best to treat on the side of dysfunction, however the opposite hand can be used to reinforce the treatment.

From the tip of the middle finger to the first knuckle=head and face
From the first knuckle to the second knuckle=neck and throat
The second knuckle to the third knuckle= chest

Ring finger
From the tip of the finger to the first knuckle=hand, first knuckle being the wrist
From the first knuckle to the second knuckle=arm, with second knuckle being elbow
From the second knuckle to the third=upper arm, with third knuckle being shoulder

Little finger
From the tip of the finger to the first knuckle=foot, first knuckle being the ankle
From the first knuckle to second=lower leg, second knuckle being the knee
From the second knuckle to the third=thigh, third knuckle being the hip

Index finger (supporting side)
From the tip of the finger to first knuckle=hand, first knuckle being the wrist
From the first knuckle to the second knuckle=arm, with second knuckle being elbow
From the second knuckle to the third=upper arm, with third knuckle being shoulder

Thumb (supporting side)
Thumb represents the anterior side of the lower extremity of the opposite side of the body.
Tip of thumb to first joint=foot, with first joint being the ankle
From the first knuckle to the second= lower leg, second knuckle being the knee
From second knuckle to base of thumb (junction of wrist and thumb)=thigh with the base of the thumb being the hip

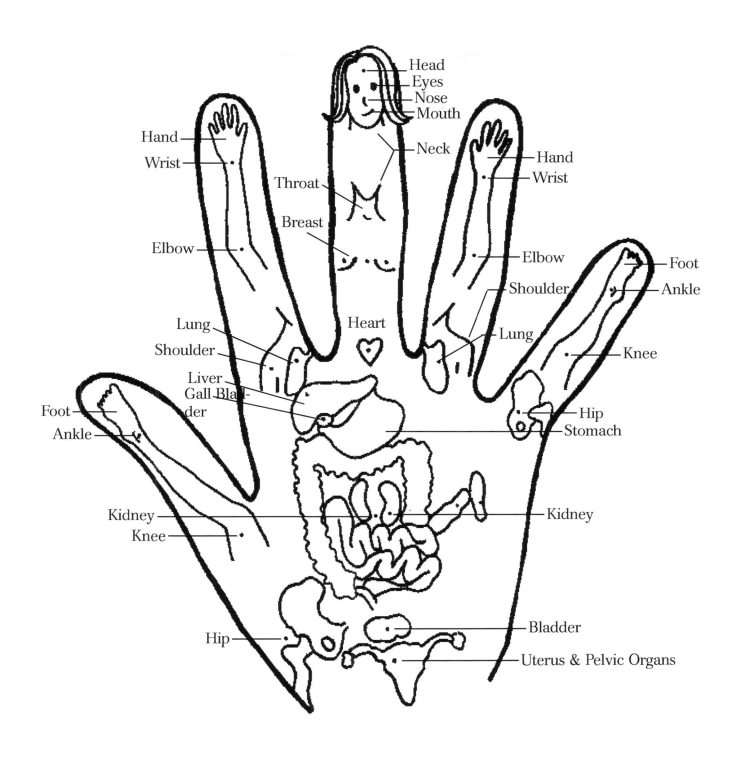

PALM OF HAND

125

PROCEDURE

Determine area of pain in the body, then search with your finger tips with a probe or with an electro search current for the tender point which corresponds to the area of dysfunction. Corresponding points are points without obvious acupuncture associations that are associated on the fingers and joints with areas on the body. Points on the fingers may also have direct correspondence to points on the body meridians and they have more of an energetic effect.

With the electro search mode, the meter reading will register higher than to the surrounding area and there will be marked tenderness on the active point. To determine the most effective treatment choose the hand on the same side as the pain. When the corresponding point on the hand is found then electrically stimulate that point with 5 Hz, 10–20 microamps, gentle wave slope for 20 seconds. Since there will usually be more than one point it is important to search out each point corresponding to the condition being treated.

Following the treatment procedure we have found it effective to place a silver pellet on the point just treated. You can determine the effectiveness of the treatment by rechecking the patients area of pain or discomfort to see if there is a reduction of symptoms.

If there is no change in symptoms, it is probable that you have not found the point that corresponds to the symptoms. It is then necessary to recheck the points or check the opposite hand's corresponding points. If there is still a symptomatic situation, it then becomes necessary to check the corresponding meridians in which the problem is associated. Example: If the patient presents with stiffness and pain in the cervical spine and after using the corresponding points the pain still exists, then look to the meridians associated with the cervical spine. We know that it is possible for the small intestine to cause a decrease in cervical rotation so you would then search the small intestine meridian on the hand for active points or determine whether that meridian should be tonified or sedated.

Examples of corresponding points:

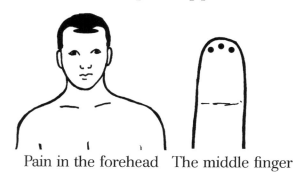

Pain in the forehead   The middle finger

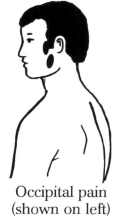

Occipital pain
(shown on left)

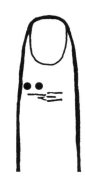

The middle finger
of the left hand

BASIC THERAPY

Basic therapy is a fundamental approach to strengthen the effects of meridian balancing or the effects of the corresponding point procedures described earlier in this chapter. When treating conditions which indicate regional or systemic weaknesses which might be determined to be visceral in origin, or which may be occurring due to reactions of other problems such as vertebral subluxations, prolonged meridian dysfunctions, trauma, diseases, and nutritional imbalances. It is effective to treat the basic areas which correspond to the patient's complaints.

In traditional Chinese medicine, we consider the organs within a specific area that need to be supported. These areas are considered zones and are referred to as Jiao. There are three Jiao: Upper, Middle, and Lower. Jiao is synonymous in reference with Upper, Middle, and Lower Heater.

Area Influenced by
Upper (Jiao) Heater

Area Influenced by
Middle (Jiao) Heater

Area Influenced by
Lower (Jiao) Heater

Disorders of the head, neck, chest, heart, lung, and upper extremities are considered to be within the Upper Jiao and will be treated with points corresponding to the Upper Heater.

Disorders arising from the stomach, spleen, liver, gallbladder and trunk are of the Middle Jiao and will be treated with points of the Middle Heater.

Disorders affecting the kidney, bladder, intestine, genital and reproductive system, the pelvic region and lower extremities are within the Lower Jiao and will be treated with points of the Lower Heater.

Besides the three Jiao areas, there are also points that will benefit specific areas of the body.

Other Hand Points (charts follow)

Abdominal basic points : Treat any problem within the abdominal area. These points overlap the Upper and Lower Heaters.

Neural basic points: These points are helpful in conditions involving the nervous system including emotional and neuropathic problems of somatic nature.

Lumbar basic points: The lower back is one of the most common areas of complaint and many times it is associated with the Bladder and Gallbladder meridians. Lumbar basic points treat these areas.

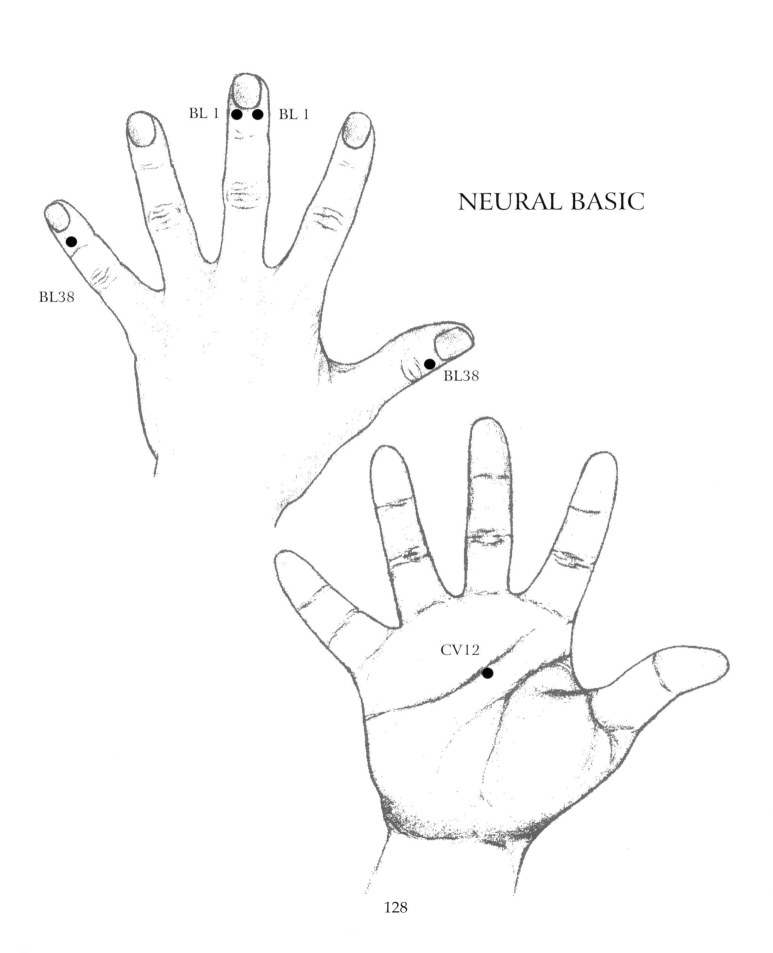

NEURAL BASIC

BL 1
BL 1
BL38
BL38
CV12

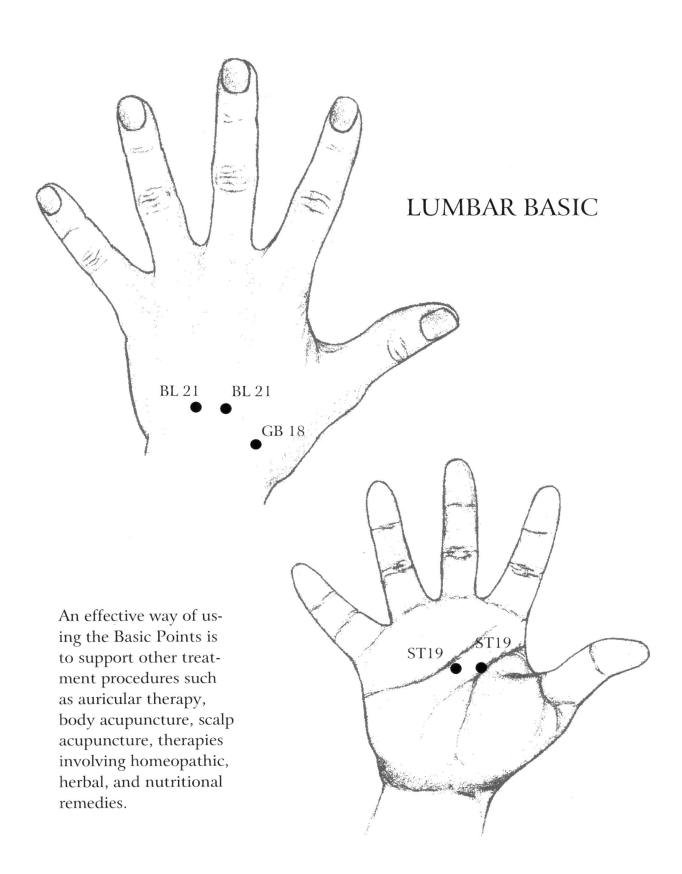

LUMBAR BASIC

BL 21   BL 21

GB 18

ST19   ST19

An effective way of using the Basic Points is to support other treatment procedures such as auricular therapy, body acupuncture, scalp acupuncture, therapies involving homeopathic, herbal, and nutritional remedies.

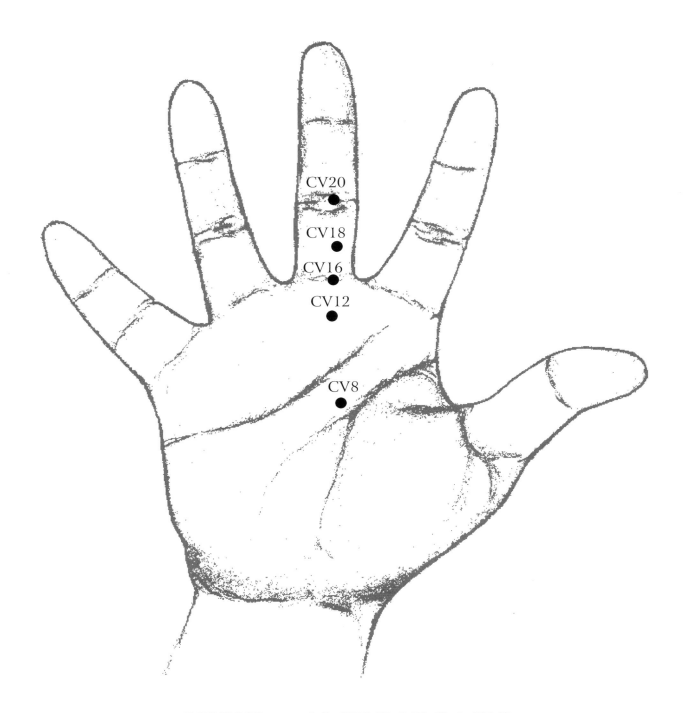

UPPER and MIDDLE BASIC
(Upper Heater is CV 12-CV 20;
Middle Heater is CV 12- CV 8)

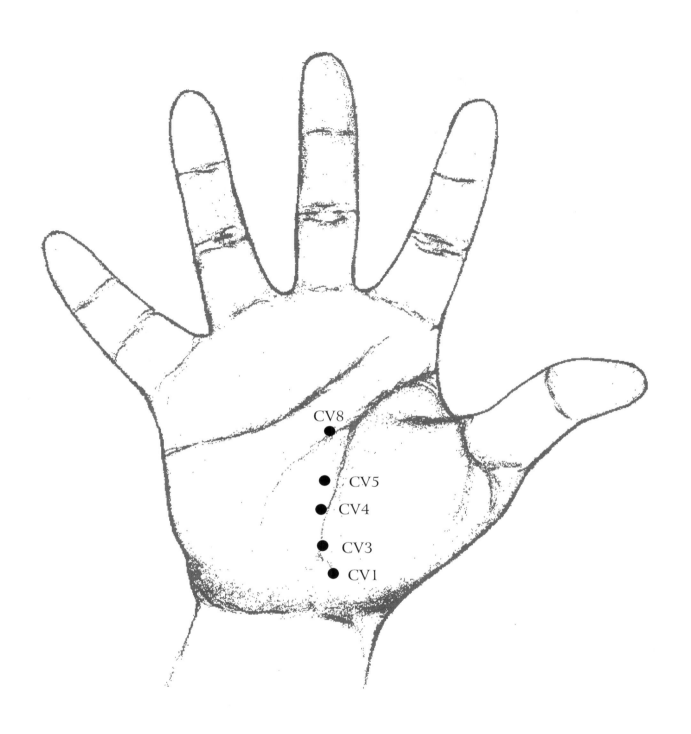

LOWER BASIC
(Lower Heater)

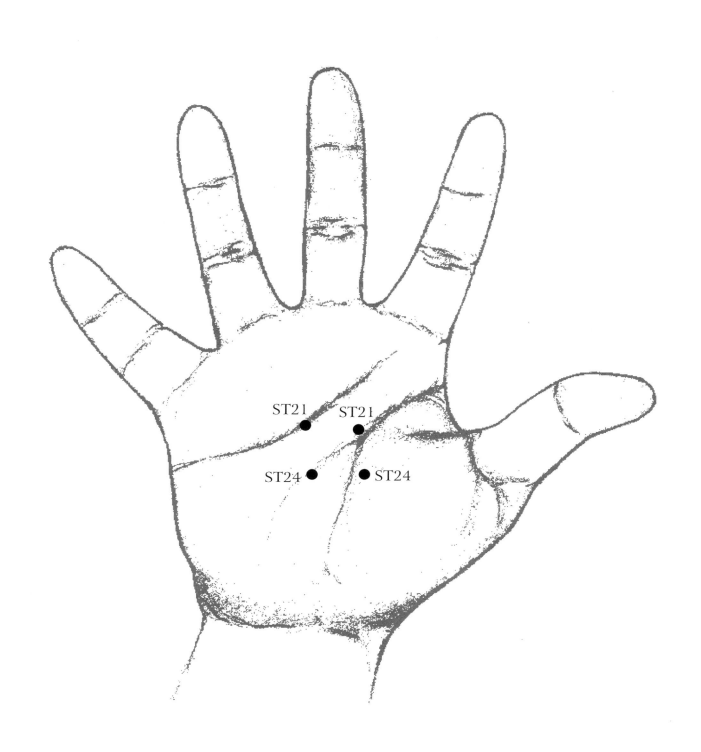

ABDOMEN BASIC

USING BASIC POINTS

To use Basic Points, correspond the Basic Points to the organs and tissues involved in the Upper, Middle, and Lower Jiao. Use 5–10 Hz, negative polarity, 40 μA, moderate Waveslope, and 20 seconds per point or till maximum response is achieved.

BALANCING MERIDIANS WITH HAND POINTS

It is important when doing any acupuncture procedure to first establish the energetic terrain which means being sure that the energy is flowing through each meridian without excess or deficiency. The same principles apply to balancing meridians with hand points as with body points.

To balance meridians:

1. Take a standard Akabane readout.

2. Determine the imbalances, looking for deficient and excessive energy levels (10 points or more).

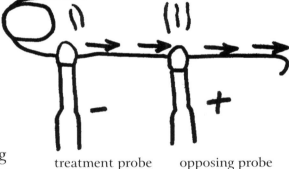

treatment probe   opposing probe

3. Tonify the most deficient yin meridian by cooperating with the natural energy flow, which is from the lowest number to the highest number on the hand meridian. Switch the Polarity to Negative. This makes the treatment probe negative and the opposing probe positive. Electricity flows from the negative to the positive.
Place the treatment probe on the lower number and the opposing probe on a higher number on the meridian at least a knuckle apart. On the hand the joints have the strongest influence on energy flow in the meridians.

4. Excessive meridians may be sedated by putting the negative probe on the highest number and the positive on the lowest number.

5. For sustained treatment following electro-stimulation and tonification, use a silver pellet on the low number and a gold pellet on the high number.

For the above procedures use the following settings:

Frequency: .5–5 Hz
Current: 10–20 μA
Polarity: Negative
Waveslope: Gentle
Time: 15–20 seconds per point.

8. When most of the meridian readings on a chart are above 75, the patient energy
    is excessive and usually the patient feels agitated or totally fatigued. It is necessary
    to drain some of the energy off. This can be done by stimulating the corresponding
    point for the skull (on posterior of first knuckle of middle finger).

    For the above procedure use the following settings:

Frequency: 5 Hz
Current: 100–200 μA
Polarity: Bi-phasic
Waveslope: Gentle
Time: Stimulate until the reading on the point is between 50 and 65.
                Then rechart. If energy doesn't come down immediately, wait about
                five minutes, then recheck.

KOREAN HAND ACUPOINT THERAPY MERIDIAN CHARTS

The following charts show the acupoints for the hand meridians. You will see that the
numbers are not always consecutive. There are also numbers missing. This is because
some points are not numbered in order and some are insignificant and have been omitted
for clarity. There is a Kidney 1 chart, but not one for Kidney 2. For the therapy procedures described in this section, only Kidney 1 has any significance.

LUNG

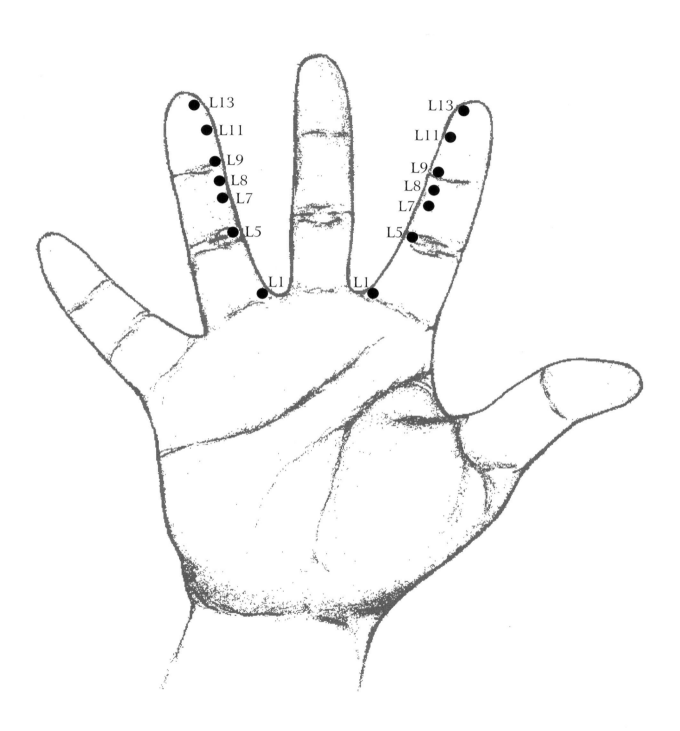

LARGE INTESTINE

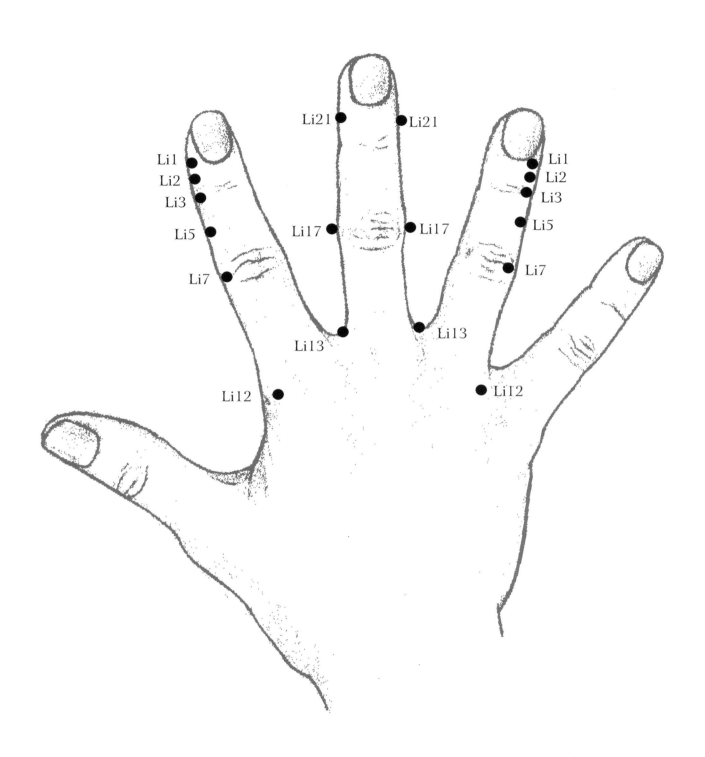

TRIPLE WARMER

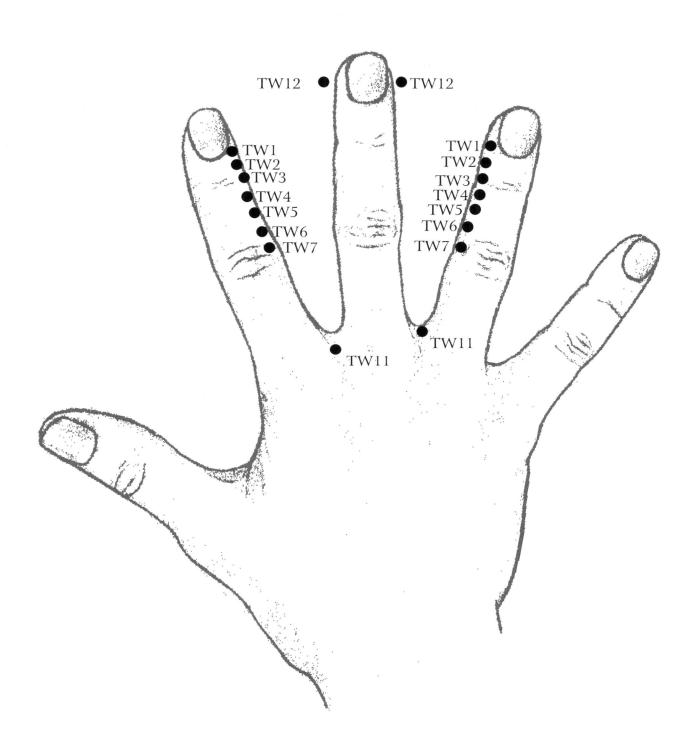

HEART CONSTRICTOR

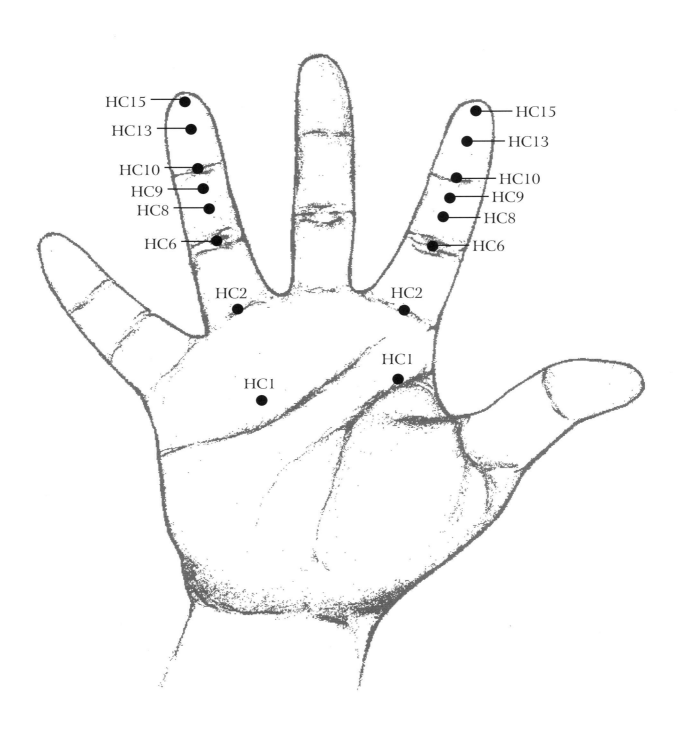

HC15
HC13
HC10
HC9
HC8
HC6
HC2
HC1

HC15
HC13
HC10
HC9
HC8
HC6
HC2
HC1

HEART

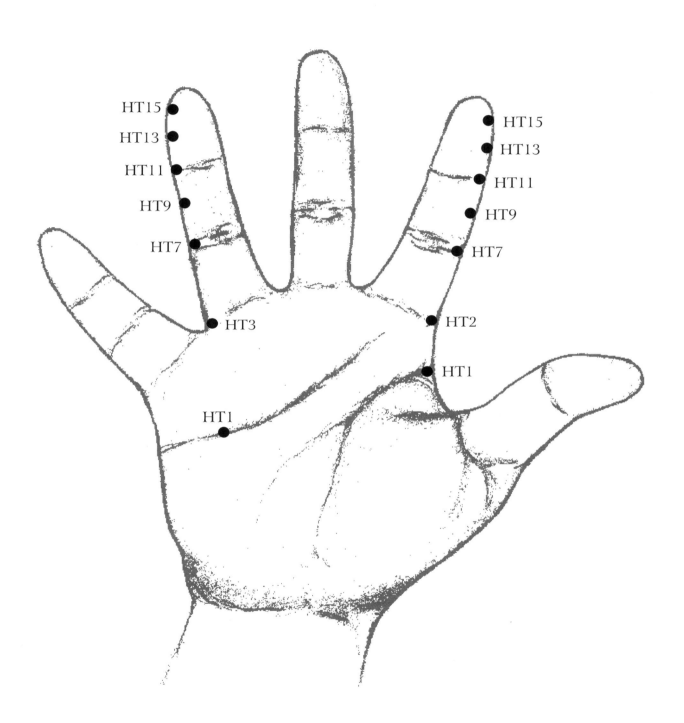

SMALL INTESTINE

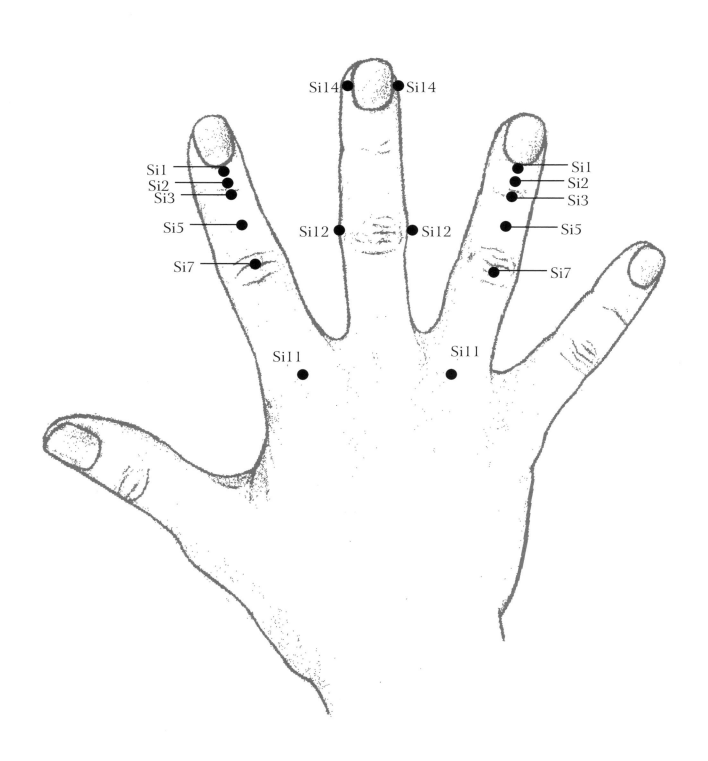

SPLEEN

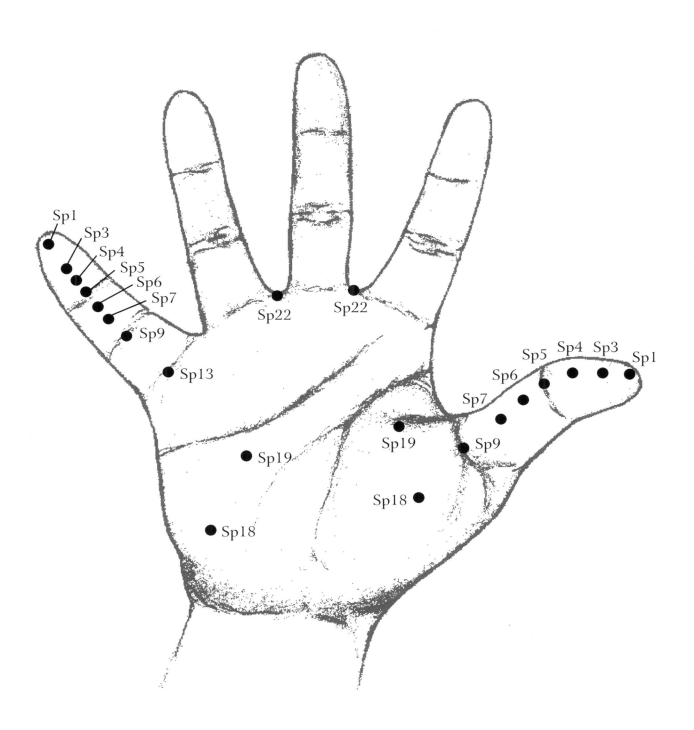

141

STOMACH

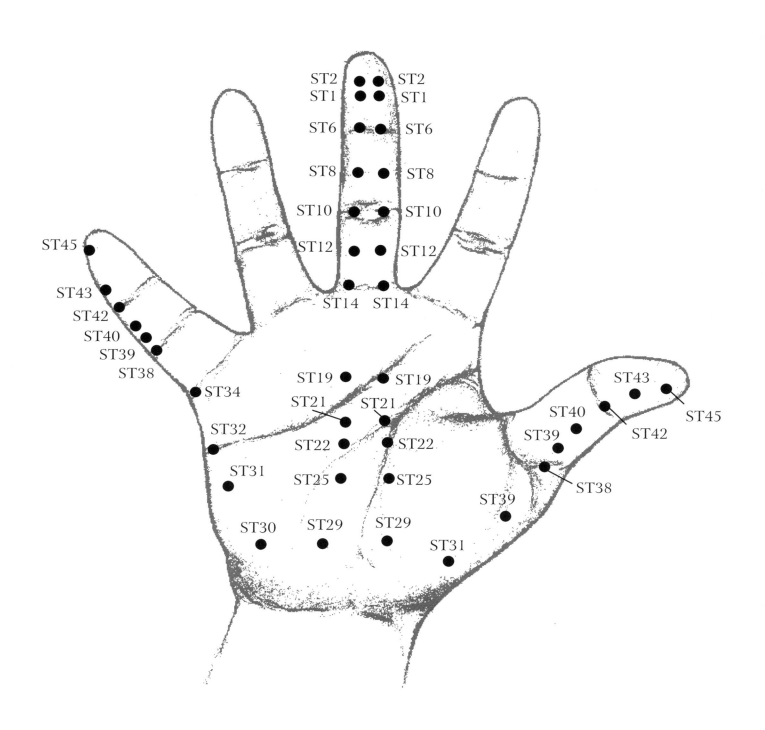

LIVER

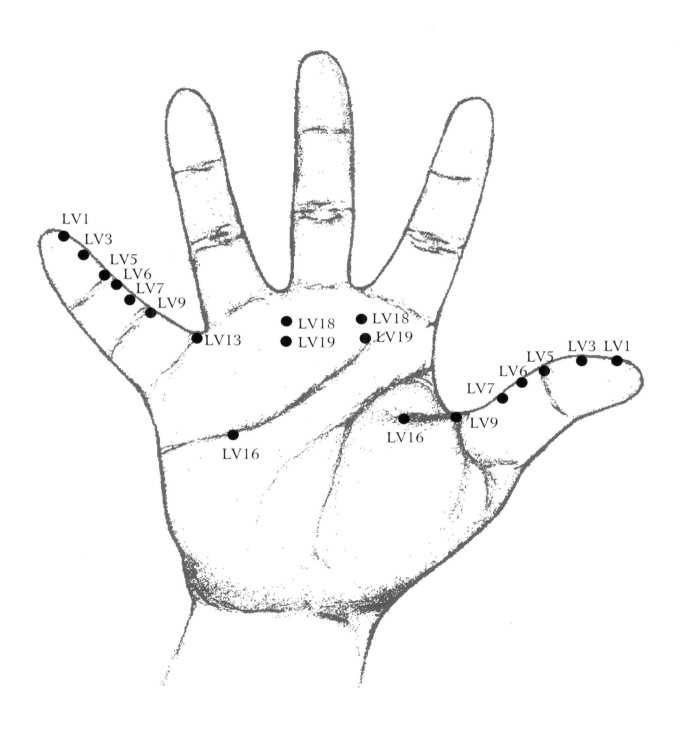

GALLBLADDER

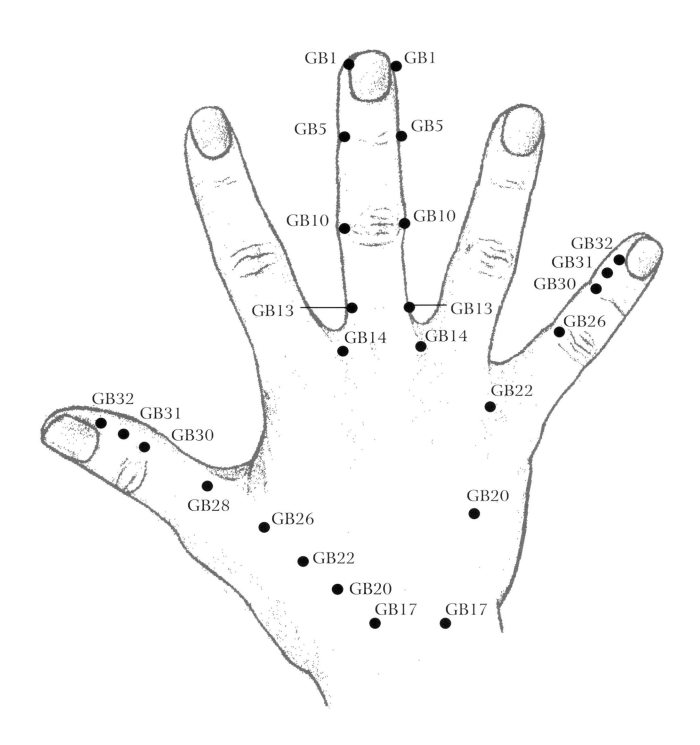

KIDNEY I

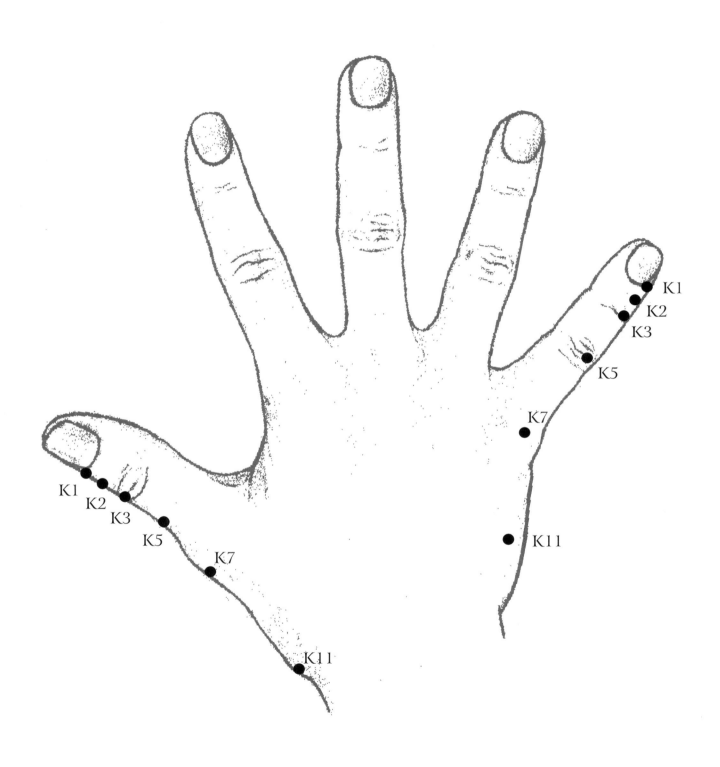

145

BLADDER

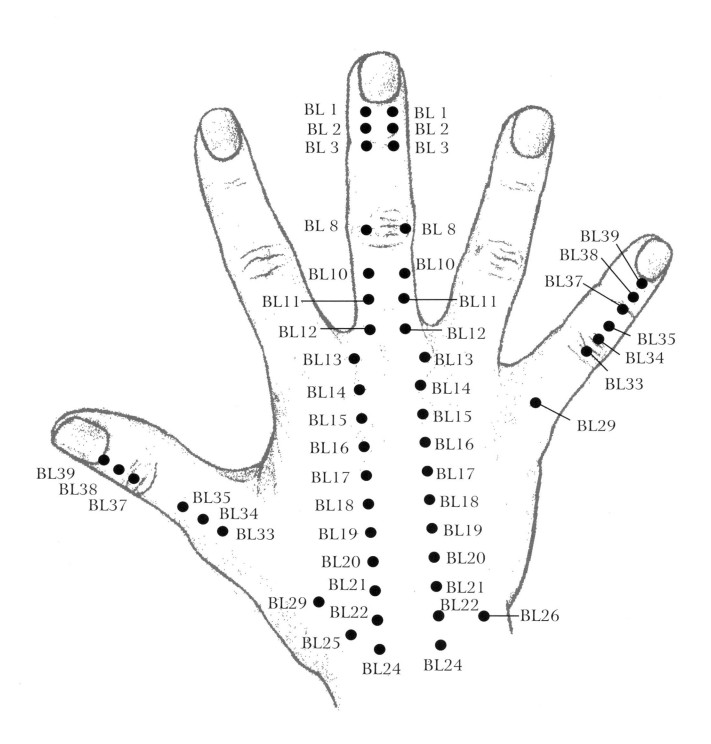

CONCEPTION VESSEL

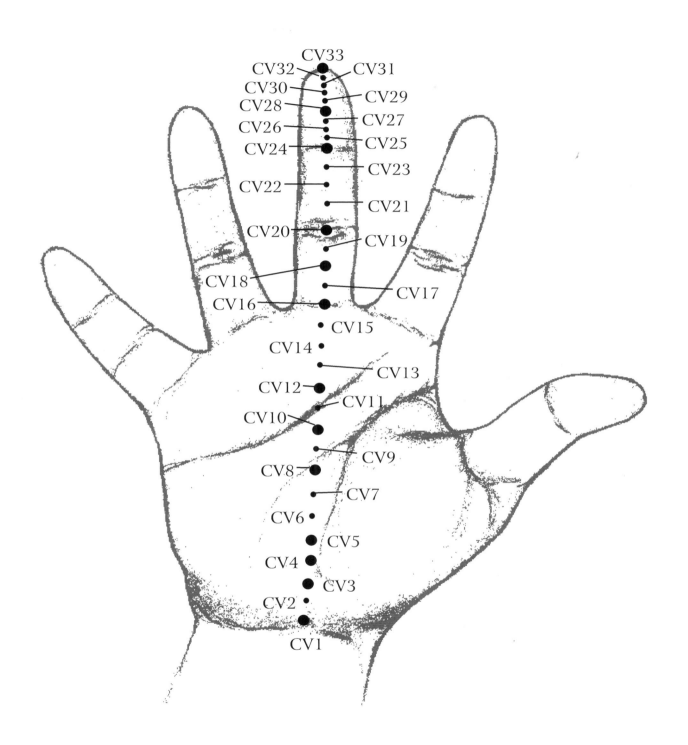

GOVERNING VESSEL

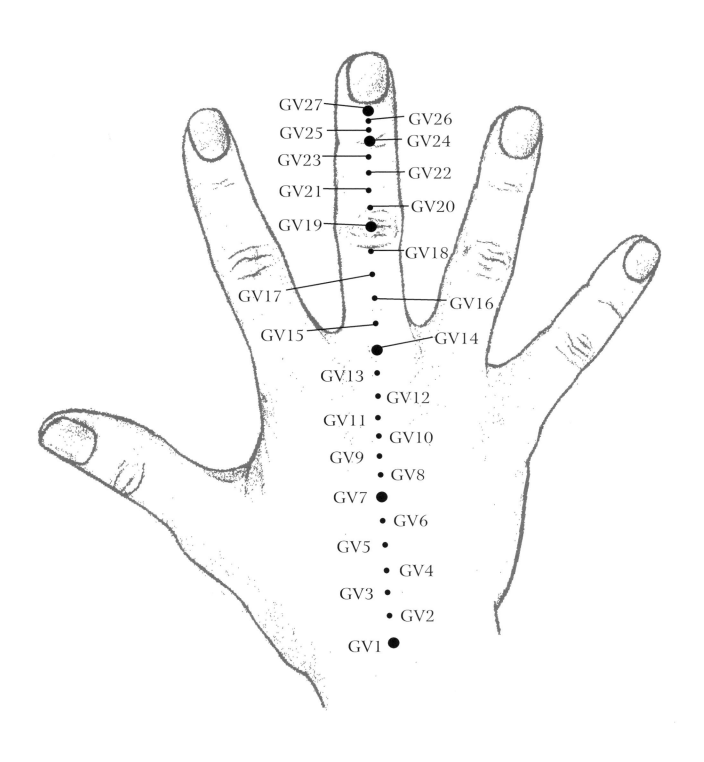

GV27 • GV26
GV25 • GV24
GV23 • GV22
GV21 • GV20
GV19 • GV18
GV17 •
GV15 • GV16
GV14
GV13 •
• GV12
GV11 •
• GV10
GV9 •
• GV8
GV7 •
• GV6
GV5 •
• GV4
GV3 •
• GV2
GV1 •

CHARTING MERIDIANS USING HAND SOURCE POINTS

It is also possible to do a meridian readout by measuring the Source Points on the microsystem of the hand. The Source Point readout is similar to the Ryodo-Raku readout in body acupuncture. This readout is more like measuring the organ response than the energetic flow through the meridians which is what the Akabane readout indicates.

Information received when charting the hand system is primarily similar to that which is received when charting for Ryodo-Raku. They both use Source Points, however Ryodo-Raku uses Source Points on the wrists and ankles and hand acupuncture Source Points are located on the ring and little finger of each hand. It is necessary to measure the twelve Source Points on both hands.

The Source Points for the yin meridians are located on the palmer side of the fingers. The Source Points for the yang meridians are located on the backs of the fingers.

To chart Source Points, search Source Points on the yin meridians beginning with ST4 on the left hand and then the Source Points on the right hand. Record each reading when the meter stabilizes. Write the number of the reading in the box under the appropriate meridian and side of the body. Then search and record the yang points on each hand, starting with KI 3 on the left.

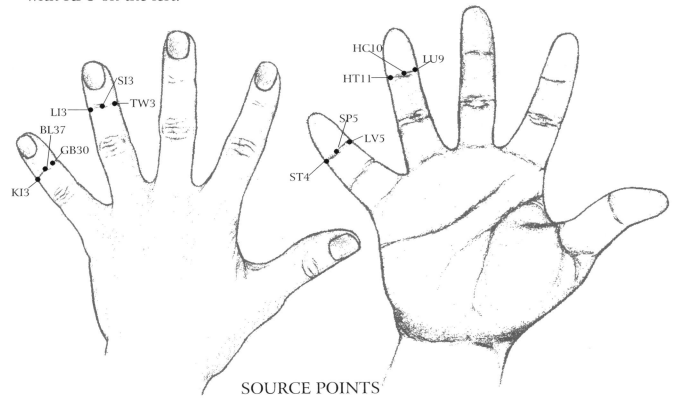

SOURCE POINTS

BALANCING MERIDIANS WITH HAND POINTS

~ Dysbalance in meridians is indicated by differences in meter readings of more than 8 points between right and left sides of the body or between coupled meridians.

~ To tonify a meridian stimulate with the energy flow. Use the negative probe on a lower number on the meridian and the positive probe on the higher number on the meridian as described on p.133.
> Examples:
> LU: to tonify place positive on LU 11, negative on LU 5
> LI: to tonify, place positive on LI 7, negative on LI 3

~ To sedate a meridian, stimulate against the energy flow as described on p. 133.
> Examples:
> LI: to sedate, place negative on LI 7, positive on LI 3
> LU: to sedate, place negative on LU 11, positive on LU 5

~ To reinforce the electrical stimulation, place a silver ion pellet on the point with the lower number and a gold on the point with the higher number.

~ To support sedation, use the silver pellet on the point with the higher number and gold on the point with the lower number.

Instrument Settings:	
Frequency:	.5–5 Hz
Current:	10–20 μA
Polarity:	Negative
Waveslope:	Gentle
Time:	15–20 seconds

~ Follow using corresponding and basic points associated with patient's symptoms.

MISCELLANEOUS

COMMON POINT TREATMENT INDICATIONS

LU 7   headache, stiff neck, cough, asthma, facial paralysis

LI 4   headache, toothache, tonsillitis, rhinitis, pharyngitis, opthalmalgia, facial paralysis, simple thyroid goiter, pain and paralysis of the upper extremities, arthritis of mandible, hyperhydrosis, hypohydrosis, common cold with fever

LI 11   pain in shoulder and arm, paralysis of upper extremities, fever, hypertension, chorea, eczema, neurodermatitis, disorder of the cubital joint and its surrounding soft tissue

ST 25   acute and chronic gastro-enteritis, dysentery, constipation, intestinal paralysis, diarrhea in children and infants, paralysis of M. abdominis, appendicitis, acute intestinal obstruction

ST 26   abdominal pain, menorrhalgia

ST 29   amenorrhea, menorrhalgia, prolapse of uterus, acute epididymitis, chronic pelvic inflammation, hernia

ST 36   gastalgia, nausea and vomiting, abdominal distention, constipation, bacillary dysentery, enteritis and diseases of the digestive tract, also for general tonic purposes

ST 40   cough, excessive sputum, dizziness and vertigo, schizophrenia, epilepsy, paralysis and numbness of lower extremities, hemiplegia, dyspepsia

SP 6   borborygmus, abdominal distention, loose stool, irregular menstruation, nocturnal emission, impotence, spermatorrhea, orchitis, enuresis, frequency of urination, retention of urine, hemiplegia, neurasthenia

SP 9   abdominal distention, edema, dysuria, enuresis, nocturnal emission, irregular menstruation, dysentery

SP10   irregular menstruation, functional uterine bleeding, urticaria

HT 3   numbness of hand and arm, tremor of forearm, angina pectoris, disorders of the cubital joint and its surrounding soft tissue

HT 6	neurasthenia, angina pectoris, palpitation, night sweating
HT 7	dream-disturbed sleep, insomnia, anxiety, palpitation, hysteria
SI 3	stiffness or rigidity of neck, tinnitus, deafness, occipital headache, lumbago, paralysis of upper extremities, night sweating, epilepsy, malaria
SI 4	arthritis of the elbow, wrist, and finger joints, headache, tinnitus, vomiting, cholecystitis
BL 13	cough, dyspnea, pulmonary tuberculosis, pneumonia, lesion of the soft tissue of the back
BL 38	cystitis, constipation, dysuresis, paralysis of lateral aspect of lower extremities
BL 54	cystitis, hemorrhoids, sciatica, paralysis and numbness or pain of lower extremities
BL 60	painful heel, weakness or paralysis of lower extremities
KI 1	coma, shock, mania, hysteria, epilepsy, infantile convulsion, unchecked nausea and vomiting, sore throat, dysuresis, also vertical headache
KI 4	neurasthenia, hysteria, hemoptysis, asthma, dysuresis, constipation, painful heel
KI 27	chest pain, cough, asthma, vomiting
HC 6	vomiting, gastralgia, insomnia, palpitation, angian pectoris, hysteria, epilepsy, pain in the chest and costal region, hiccough (spasm of diaphragm)
HC 7	insomnia, palpitation, epilepsy, disorders of the wrist joint and its surrounding soft tissue
TH 2	headache, conjunctivitis, deafness, sore throat, pain in hand and arm, malaria
TH 3	deafness, tinnitus, headache, sore throat and paralysis of upper extremities or hands
TH 5	paralysis of the upper extremities, thoraco-costal pain, headache, deafness, tinnitus, stiff neck, common cold, fever

GB 20   common cold, headache, dizziness and vertigo, stiffness of neck, hypertension, tinnitus

GB 21   pain in shoulder and back, rigidity and stiffness of neck, motor impairment of upper extremities, mastitis, hyperthyroidism, functional uterine bleeding

GB 30   sciatica, paralysis of lower extremities, disorders of the hip joint and its surrounding soft tissue

GB 34   hemiplegia, diseases of the gall bladder, lumbago and leg pain, dizziness and vertigo, acid regurgitation

GB 39   paralysis of lower extremities, stiffness and rigidity of neck, disorders of the ankle joint and its surrounding soft tissue

GB 40   pain in lower extremities, pain in ankle joint, thoracalgia

GB 43   deafness, headache, dizziness, chest pain, intercostal neuralgia

LV 2   irregular menstruation, urethritis, enuresis, pain in costal region, hypertension, epilepsy, insomnia, redness and swelling of eye

LV 3   headache, dizziness, epilepsy, convulsions in children and infants, eye diseases, hernia, uterine bleeding, mastitis

LV 5   inflammation of pelvic organs, retention of urine, spermatorrhea, impotence

LV 8   infection of urogenital system, spermatorrhea, impotence, hernia, disorders of the knee joint and its surrounding soft tissue

GV 20   epilepsy schizophrenia, apoplexy, headache

CV 4   spermatorrhea, impotence, menorrhalgia, irregular menstruation, diarrhea, enuresis. Also used as a tonic

CV 12   gastralgia, gastroptosis, vomiting, dyspepsia, abdominal distention

COMMON POINTS

	LU	SP	HT	KI	HC	LV	LI	ST	SI	BL	TH	GB
Wood	LU11	SP1	HT9	KI 1	HC9	LV1	LI 3	ST43	SI 3	BL65	TH3	GB41
Fire	LU10	SP2	HT8	KI 2	HC8	LV2	LI 5	ST41	SI 5	BL60	TH6	GB38
Earth	LU9	SP3	HT7	KI 6	HC7	LV3	LI 11	ST36	SI 8	BL54	TH10	GB34
Metal	LU8	SP5	HT4	KI 7	HC5	LV4	LI 1	ST45	SI 1	BL67	TH1	GB44
Water	LU5	SP9	HT3	KI10	HC3	LV8	LI 2	ST44	SI 2	BL66	TH2	GB43
Tonifi-cation	LU9	SP2	HT9	KI 7	HC9	LV8	LI 11	ST41	SI 3	BL67	TH3	GB43
Sedation	LU5	SP5	HT7	KI 1	HC7	LV2	LI 2	ST45	SI 8	BL65	TH10	GB38
Source	LU9	SP3	HT7	KI 3	HC7	LV3	LI 4	ST42	SI 4	BL64	TH4	GB40
Associ-ated	BL13	BL20	BL15	BL23	BL14	BL18	BL25	BL21	BL27	BL28	BL22	BL19
Alarm	LU1	LV13	CV14	GB25	CV17	LV14	ST25	CV12	CV4	CV3	CV5	GB24
LUO	LU7	SP4	HT5	KI 5	HC6	LV5	LI 6	ST40	SI 7	BL58	TH5	GB37
Entry	LU1	SP1	HT1	KI 1	HC1	LV1	LI 4	ST1	SI 1	BL1	TH1	GB1
Exit	LU7	SP21	HT9	KI22	HC8	LV14	LI20	ST42	SI19	BL67	TH23	GB41
Lower Meeting Point	—	—	—	—	—	—	ST37	ST36	SI39	BL54	BL53	GB34
Upper Meeting Point	—	—	—	—	—	—	LI 11	—	SI8	—	TH10	—

USING ALARM POINTS

Palpation and therapy localization of the Reflex Points on the thorax and abdomen can be used to verify diagnoses of affected meridians.

When a Reflex Point is located, press lightly with the tip of your index finger. If the patient feels pain, it indicates that the organ in question is hypoactive. If no pain is felt, press more deeply. Pain upon heavier pressure means the organ is hyperactive. If no pain is felt either way, the organ is in a state of equilibrium.

Therapy Localization, taught by Dr. George Goodheart, also uses these points. You can hold the respective points and test an indicator muscle. If light pressure causes the muscle to become weak, the meridian is hypoactive. If the weakness occurs upon deep pressure, the meridian is hyperactive.

Drs. Beardall, D.C. Rarez, D.C., and Ladd, D.C., found that they could challenge an Alarm Point and follow the superficial flow of energy as noted in the Horay Cycle, counter clockwise. Each meridian that was deficient would cause weakening of the associate muscle. But when they came to the blocked meridian, the muscle would not weaken. They would stimulate the Connecting Point and recheck the meridians clockwise to verify correction. This procedure may also be used applying the Five Elements chart and testing counter clockwise to locate the excessive energy blocks.

DESCRIPTIONS OF ALARM POINTS

LUNG   located between second rib and clavicle (LU 1, bilateral)

LARGE INTESTINE on right side of abdomen (ST 25) and corresponds to the McBurney Point

STOMACH located midway between the sternum and umbilicus (VC 12)

SPLEEN   on the tip of the 11th rib (LV 13, bilateral)

HEART   at the tip of the xiphoid process. If pain reflex to light pressure, HC is affected. Heavy pressure reflex indicates the heart is hyperactive (VC 14)

SMALL INTESTINE between the umbilicus and the pubis (VC 4)

BLADDER	above the pubis on the meridian line (VC 3)
KIDNEY	on the tip of the 12th rib (GB 25)
HEART CONSTRICTOR	on the meridian line at the level of the nipples (VC 17)
TRI HEATER	between the umbilicus on the meridian line (VC 5)
GALLBLADDER	on the lower edge of the 6th rib (GB 24, bilateral)
LIVER	on the 5th rib, about level with the nipples (LV 14, bilateral)

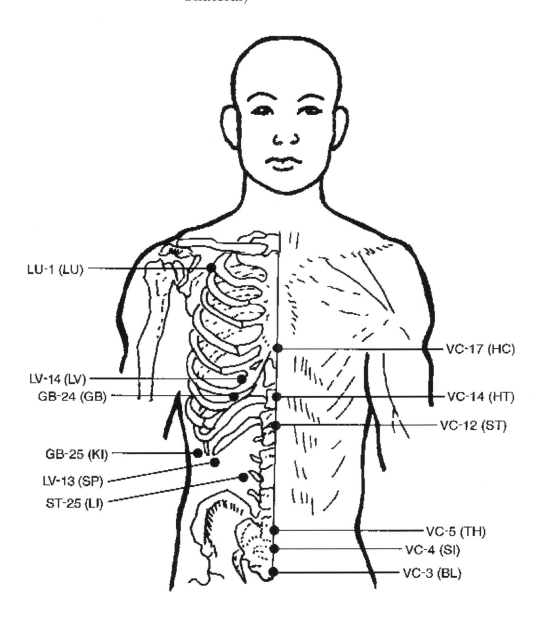

DISEASED ORGANS
AND THEIR RELATED ORGANS

According to the Chinese, when one organ is diseased, four other organs become endangered. This relationship is based upon the laws of traditional acupuncture. It is important to recognize these possibilities, both for treating and for preventive care.

DISEASED ORGAN	RELATED ORGANS
HEART	1. Small Intestine 2. Lungs 3. Gallbladder 4. Circulation
GENITO-URINARY	1. Kidney 2. Tri-Heater 3. Spleen-Pancreas 4. Stomach
CIRCULATION	1. Tri-Heater 2. Kidneys 3. Stomach 4. Small Intestine
GALLBLADDER	1. Liver 2. Stomach 3. Heart 4. Large Intestine
LUNGS	1. Large Intestine 2. Heart 3. Urinary Bladder 4. Liver

STOMACH
1. Spleen-Pancreas
2. Gallbladder
3. Circulation
4. Urinary Bladder

SMALL INTESTINE
1. Heart
2. Large Intestine
3. Liver
4. Endocrine System

KIDNEY
1. Urinary Bladder
2. Circulation-Sex
3. Large Intestine
4. Spleen-Pancreas

ENDOCRINE
1. Circulation
2. Urinary Bladder
3. Spleen-Pancreas
4. Small Intestine

LIVER
1. Gallbladder
2. Spleen-Pancreas
3. Small Intestine
4. Lung

LARGE INTESTINE
1. Lung
2. Small Intestine
3. Kidneys
4. Gallbladder

SPLEEN-PANCREAS
1. Stomach
2. Liver
3. Tri-Heater
4. Kidney

Suggested Reading

Dale, Ralph Alan, "Acupuncture Electrodiagnosis: Which Acupoints Can Most Easily Provide the Best Diagnostic Information?" *American Journal of Acupuncture, Vol 21, No. 2*, 1993; pp. 171–178.

Greenlee, Dennis L. 1995. *The Healing Ear.* Kelseyville: Earthen Vessel Productions, Inc.

Oleson, Terry. 1992. *Auriculotherapy Manual.* Los Angeles. Health Care Alternatives.

Oleson, Terry. 1995. *International Handbook of Ear Reflex Points.* Los Angeles. Health Care Alternatives.

Picker, Robert. *Current Trends: Low-Volt Pulsed Microamp Stimulation,* Parts I and II. Reprint available from Earthen Vessel Productions, Inc.

Wing, Thomas W. 1994. *Ear-Ricular Therapy* Kelseyville. Earthen Vessel Productions, Inc.

Wing, Thomas W. 1986. *Reprints Vol. I.* Kelseyville. Earthen Vessel Productions, Inc.

Wing, Thomas W. 1994. *Reprints Vol. 2.* Kelseyville. Earthen Vessel Productions, Inc.

Made in the USA
Middletown, DE
03 March 2022

62037804R00095